The Periodontic Syllabus

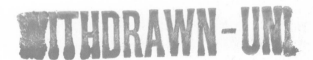

The Periodontic Syllabus

Edited by

PETER F. FEDI, JR., D.D.S., M.Sc.

Rinehart Professor of Dentistry
Director of Clinical Specialties
Director of Advanced Education Programs
School of Dentistry
University of Missouri–Kansas City
Kansas City, Missouri

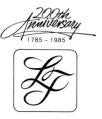

Lea & Febiger   *1985   Philadelphia*

Lea & Febiger
600 Washington Square
Philadelphia, PA 19106-4198
U.S.A.
(215) 922-1330

Library of Congress Cataloging in Publication Data
Main entry under title:

The Periodontic syllabus.

  Rev. ed. of: Periodontics syllabus [2nd ed.] 1975.
  Includes bibliographies and index.
  1. Periodontal diseases—Outlines, syllabi, etc.
I. Fedi, Peter F. II. Periodontics syllabus. [DNLM:
1. Periodontal Diseases. WU 240 P4473]
RK361.P462 1985   617.6′32   84-27787
ISBN 0-8121-0982-1

PRINTED IN THE UNITED STATES OF AMERICA

Print No. 4 3 2 1

Preface

The value of a syllabus is its ability to remain current. Whereas textbooks, due to their complexity and comprehensiveness, have a tendency to become obsolete in a relatively short time, a syllabus can be readily corrected and brought up to date simply and rapidly. This need for revision is especially important in the field of periodontics, in which therapeutic concepts are so dynamic and undergo rapid change.

The purpose of this syllabus is really twofold. First we wanted to update the syllabus that we have been using these past few years, and second, to offer to the student, whether a predoctoral or a continuing student, a manual that can be used in "cookbook fashion" that logically explains therapeutic concepts based primarily on biologic principles. The *Syllabus* is not meant to be a textbook; in fact, it should complement current textbooks that deliver indepth knowledge of the basics. Understandably, there are a few chapters that briefly review the basic concepts of biologic science, which may be repetitious to the predoctoral student. We feel, however, that these chapters review the current concepts for the busy general practitioner who has been unable to keep up to date in the area of the biologic sciences. This syllabus, after all, is directed toward the generalist who must assume the responsibility of diagnosing, treating,

and referring patients with periodontal problems. The generalist in today's dental arena must have the knowledge and skills to practice holistic dentistry. The treatment of periodontal problems must, therefore, become an integral part of every general practice.

This publication is basically a revision of the periodontics syllabus prepared by members of the faculty in the Department of Periodontics at the Naval Graduate Dental School, Bethesda, Maryland. The first edition was written by Dr. Perry Alexander in 1960. His syllabus was revised in 1964 and 1967 by Drs. Peter Fedi and Corry Holmes. For the 1968 edition, Dr. Fedi requested and received help in revision from Drs. Joseph Lawrence, Sam Holroyd, William Moffitt, and Jefferson Hardin.

The most popular edition, however, was published in 1975 and was authored by Dr. Gerald Bowers, assisted by Drs. Joseph Lawrence and John E. Williams. This version has sold thousands of copies all over the world, but it is now out of print. The demand remains and therefore we make this effort to publish a new edition of a Navy tradition. This syllabus, therefore, is dedicated to all the pioneers of Navy periodontics who have contributed to the high esteem now held for the Navy Dental Corps in the field of periodontics.

Kansas City, Missouri

PETER F. FEDI, JR.

v

Contributors

Peter F. Fedi, Jr., D.D.S., M.Sc.
Rinehart Professor of Dentistry
Director of Clinical Specialties
Director of Advanced Education
Programs
School of Dentistry
University of Missouri-Kansas City
Kansas City, Missouri

Jefferson F. Hardin, D.D.S., M.S.
Associate Professor
Department of Periodontics
School of Dentistry
Medical College of Georgia
Augusta, Georgia

William J. Killoy, D.D.S., M.S.
Professor and Chairman
Department of Periodontics
School of Dentistry
University of Missouri-Kansas City
Kansas City, Missouri

Joseph J. Lawrence, D.D.S., M.S.
Professor and Chairman
Department of Periodontics
School of Dentistry
Louisiana State University
New Orleans, Louisiana

Herman D. Tow, D.D.S., M.S.
Professor and Chairman
Department of Periodontics
University of Oklahoma College of
Dentistry
Oklahoma City, Oklahoma

Arthur R. Vernino, D.D.S.
Professor
Department of Periodontics
University of Oklahoma College of
Dentistry
Oklahoma City, Oklahoma

John E. Williams, D.D.S., M.S.
Associate Professor
Department of Periodontics
School of Dentistry
Indiana University
Indianapolis, Indiana

Raymond A. Yukna, D.M.D., M.S.
Clinical Professor of Periodontics
Department of Periodontics
School of Dentistry
Louisiana State University
New Orleans, Louisiana
Clinical Professor of Surgical
Dentistry
School of Dentistry
University of Colorado
Denver, Colorado

Contents

CHAPTER 1

The Periodontium

GINGIVA

Terminology

The gingiva is composed of keratinizing epithelium and connective tissue. The following terminology is used when describing the gingiva (Fig. 1–1).

1. *Marginal (free) gingiva.* The portion of the gingiva surrounding the neck of the tooth, not directly attached to the tooth, and forming the soft tissue wall of the gingival sulcus. It extends from the free gingival margin to the free gingival groove.
2. *Free gingival groove.* The shallow line or depression on the surface of the gingiva dividing the free gingiva from the attached gingiva. The free gingival groove often but not always corresponds to the location of the bottom of the gingival sulcus.
3. *Keratinized gingiva.* The band of keratinized gingiva from free gingival margin to the mucogingival junction (Fig. 1–1).

The width of the keratinized gingiva varies from less than 1 to 9 mm. Teeth that are prominent in the arch, such as the mandibular canine and premolars, frequently have a narrow zone of keratinized gingiva. High frenum and high muscle attachments are likewise associated with a narrow width of keratinized gingiva. Often patients who maintain healthy keratinized gingiva have less than 1 mm of attached gingiva. If there is no band of attached gingiva, however, and extension of the lip or cheek results in a pull on the free gingival margin, an increased susceptibility to tissue breakdown may result. An adequate width of attached gingiva may then be defined as the amount of tissue necessary to assist in maintaining the gingival margin in a stable position and in a state of health.

4. *Attached gingiva.* The portion of the gingiva that extends apically from the area of the free gingival groove to the mucogingival junction. In the absence of inflammation, the attached gingiva is clearly defined, except in the hard palate, where there is no clinical demarcation between the attached gingiva and the remaining masticatory mucosa. The attached gingiva is normally covered by keratinized or parakeratinized epithelium that has marked rete ridges extending into the connective tissue. There is no submucosa, and the attached gingiva is bound tightly down to the underlying tooth and bone. It is apparent that this part of the gingiva is designed to withstand the rigors of mastication, toothbrushing, and other functional stresses.
5. *Mucogingival junction.* The scal-

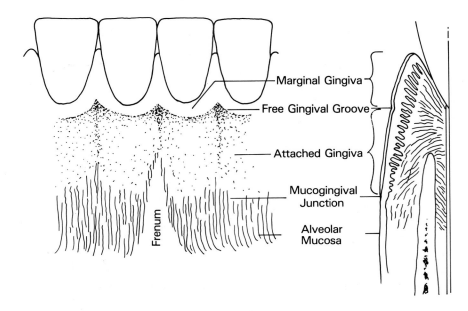

Marginal Gingiva

Free Gingival Groove

Attached Gingiva

Mucogingival Junction

Alveolar Mucosa

Frenum

Fig. 1–1.

HEALTH

DISEASE

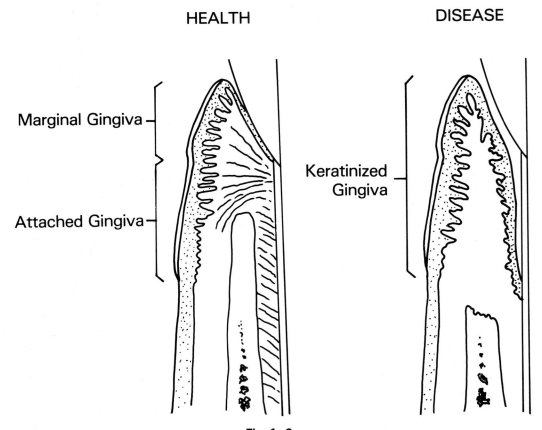

Marginal Gingiva

Attached Gingiva

Keratinized Gingiva

Fig. 1–2.

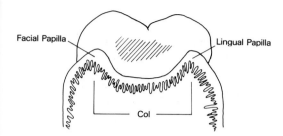

Fig. 1–3.

loped line dividing the keratinized gingiva from the alveolar mucosa (Fig. 1–2).

6. *Interdental groove.* The vertical groove, parallel to the long axes of adjacent teeth, found in the interdental area of the attached gingiva.

7. *Interdental papilla.* The portion of the gingiva that fills the interproximal space between adjacent teeth. The interdental papilla is concave, faciolingually. The saddle-like depression has been referred to as the col (Fig. 1–3).

8. *Gingival sulcus (crevice).* The space bounded by the tooth and the free gingiva, and having the junctional epithelium as its base.

Epithelium

Gingival epithelium is of the stratified squamous type. It is parakeratinized or keratinized, except for that portion lining the gingival sulcus.

Lamina Propria

This term is used to describe the connective tissue component of the gingiva. Like other tissues of the body, it consists of cells (fibroblasts, mesenchymal cells, mast cells, and macrophages), formed elements (collagenous fibers), ground substance (a polysaccharide-protein complex), and a neurovascular network. For the most part, the collagenous connective tissue fibers are oriented into coarse bundles, which are grouped according to location and direction, and are sometimes

GINGIVAL GROUP

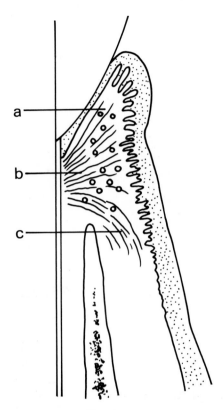

Fig. 1–4.

referred to as the gingival fiber apparatus.

Gingival Fiber Apparatus

1. *Gingival group.* These fibers extend from the cementum in three groups (termed a, b, and c) and represent the bulk of the lamina propria facially and lingually (Fig. 1–4).

2. *Circular group.* This group encompasses the teeth from the margin of the gingiva to the alveolar crest (Fig. 1–5).

3. *Transseptal group.* These fibers extend interdentally from the cementum of one tooth to that of the adjacent tooth. Some authors classify this fiber group with the principal

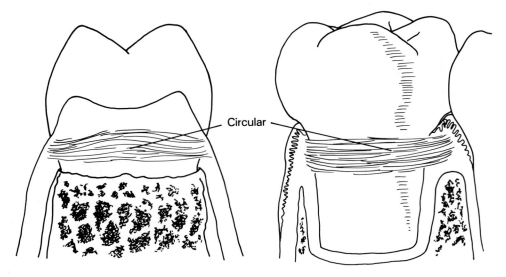

Fig. 1–5.

fibers of the periodontium rather than with the gingival fiber apparatus (Fig. 1–6).

The basic function of the gingival fiber apparatus is to maintain the free gingiva and junctional epithelium in close approximation to the tooth.

Alveolar Mucosa

The epithelium of the alveolar mucosa is thin and nonkeratinized and lacks distinct rete ridges. The connective tissue consists of a thin lamina propria and a vascular submucosal layer. The predominant connective tissue fibers are elastic; therefore, unlike the attached gingiva, the alveolar mucosa is bound loosely to the underlying periosteum of the alveolar process. Clinically, the gingiva and alveolar mucosa are separated by the mucogingival junction. On the facial aspects of the maxillary and mandibular arches, the alveolar mucosa extends to the vestibular fornix. On the lingual aspect of the mandibular arch, the arrangement is similar, but there is no demarcation in the maxillary arch. In the maxillary arch, the gingiva blends with the palatal mucosa, which is dense and firmly attached to the

underlying periosteum. It should be emphasized that the alveolar mucosa is not designed to withstand the forces of mastication; therefore, it cannot serve as gingival tissue.

Clinically Healthy Gingiva

Several terms used in describing the gingival tissues are important. A concept of what is clinically healthy will enable one to recognize what is abnormal during an examination of the gingiva. The following terms are used most often to describe normal gingiva.

1. *Color.* Normal gingiva is described as coral pink, but shading varies widely among individuals. The presence of melanin-containing cells (melanocytes) is considered normal for certain ethnic groups, e.g., Filipino, Chinese, and black individuals.
2. *Size.* Any change in size of the gingiva is a sign of periodontal disease.
3. *Contour.* This term refers primarily to the festooned appearance of the gingiva.
4. *Consistency.* The gingiva is firm, resilient, and tightly bound to the underlying bone.

TRANSSEPTAL GROUP

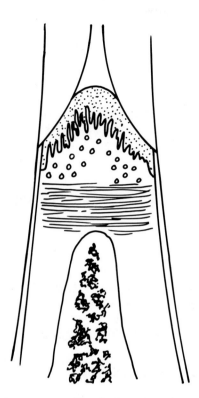

Fig. 1–6.

DENTOGINGIVAL JUNCTION

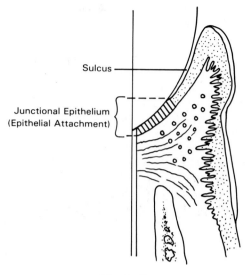

Sulcus

Junctional Epithelium
(Epithelial Attachment)

Fig. 1–7.

5. *Surface texture.* A stippled appearance is normal in the attached gingiva; loss of stippling may be a sign of periodontal disease. Stippling is caused by projections of the papillary layer of the lamina propria, which elevate the epithelium into rounded prominences that alternate with indentations of the epithelium.

6. *Tendency to bleed upon palpation or probing.* Clinically healthy gingiva will not bleed when a periodontal probe is gently inserted into the sulcus or when the marginal gingiva is palpated with the finger.

Gingival Sulcus

The gingival sulcus is lined with a nonkeratinizing, stratified squamous epithelium. The bottom of this sulcus is formed by the free surface of the junctional epithelium (Fig. 1–7). The sulcus epithelium has been likened to a semipermeable membrane through which injurious bacterial products pass into the gingiva. Tissue fluid (sulcular fluid) seeps out into the sulcus.

Junctional Epithelium (Epithelial Attachment)

This term refers to a collar-like band of nonkeratinizing basal and stratum spinosum-type cells that varies in thickness from 15 to 20 cells coronally to 1 to 2 cells apically. The cells of the junctional epithelium have relatively wider intercellular spaces and fewer desmosomes when compared with the gingival epithelium. Its location on the tooth depends on the stage of tooth eruption, but in the adult it is normally considered to be at or near the cementoenamel junction. Migration of the junctional epithelium beyond this junction is no longer considered by many dentists to be a physiologic process of aging, but rather a pathologic process, probably related to repeated plaque infection, tooth position, toothbrush trauma, etc.

The attachment of the epithelium to the tooth is comparable to the epithelial-connective tissue attachment found in skin or other body surfaces. There is a basal lamina (basement membrane) that consists of two layers: the lamina densa (adjacent to the tooth surface) and the lamina lucida, to which hemidesmosomes (attachment plaques) are attached. A sticky coating (proline and/or hydroxyproline and mucopolysaccharide), which is secreted by the epithelial cells, also binds the junctional epithelium to enamel or cementum.

Dentogingival Junction

The gingival fiber apparatus serves the important function of bracing the gingival and epithelial attachment against the surface of the tooth. The junctional epithelium and the gingival fibers act as a functional unit, the dentogingival junction (Fig. 1–7).

Blood, Lymphatic, and Nerve Supply

Gingival tissue has a rich vascular supply formed by a plexus of arterioles, capillaries, and small veins that extends from the sulcular epithelium to the outer surface of the gingiva. The blood supply of the gingiva is derived mainly from supraperiosteal branches of the internal maxillary arteries. Vessels from both the alveolar bone and the periodontal ligament merge with the supraperiosteal vessels to form the gingival plexus (Fig. 1–8).

The lymphatic drainage of the gingiva begins in the connective tissue and progresses into a network that lies external to the periosteum of the alveolar process. Lymphatic vessels drain to regional lymph nodes, particularly the submaxillary group. In addition, lymphatics beneath the epithelium extend into the periodontal ligament and accompany the blood vessels. Innervation of the gingiva comes from labial, buccal, and palatal nerves and from fibers in the periodontal ligament.

PERIODONTAL LIGAMENT

The periodontal ligament comprises the white, collagenous connective tissue fibers that surround the root of the tooth and attach to the alveolar process. There are relatively few elastic fibers in the periodontal ligament. The apparent elasticity is due to the wavy configuration of the principal fibers, which permits slight movement when the tooth is placed under stress.

Functions

The functions of the periodontal ligament are as follows.
1. It maintains the biologic activity of cementum and bone.
2. It supplies nutrients and removes waste products via blood and lymph vessels.
3. It maintains the relation of a tooth to hard and soft tissues.
4. It is capable of transmitting tactile pressure and pain sensations by the trigeminal pathway. The sense of localization is imparted through proprioceptive nerve endings.

Width

Width of the periodontal ligament space varies with age, location of the tooth, and degree of stress to which the tooth was subjected. The mesial side is thinner than the distal side, owing to the physiologic mesial drift of teeth. A tooth that is not in function has a thin periodontal ligament, with loss of direction of the principal fibers. A tooth under normal use has a thicker periodontal ligament and a normal configuration of the principal fibers. A tooth in functional occlusion has a periodontal ligament space of approximately 0.25 ± 0.10 mm. A tooth subjected to abnormal stress has a

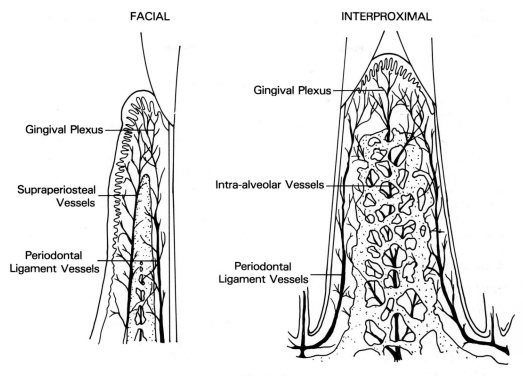

FACIAL

INTERPROXIMAL

Gingival Plexus

Suraperiosteal
Vessels

Periodontal
Ligament Vessels

Gingival Plexus

Intra-alveolar Vessels

Periodontal
Ligament Vessels

Fig. 1–8.

considerably thicker periodontal ligament space.

Blood Supply

This is derived from three sources.
1. Blood vessels entering the periodontal ligament from the apical area.
2. Interalveolar (interdental) arteries passing into the periodontal ligament from the interdental alveolar process.
3. Anastomosing vessels from the gingiva.

Nerve Supply

The nerves are both myelinated and naked. They vary from knoblike swellings to free endings between fibers. The nerve bundles follow the course of the blood vessels. Their primary purpose is to transmit proprioceptive sensations via the trigeminal pathways, which give a sense of localization when a tooth is touched.

Attachment Apparatus

The attachment apparatus comprises alveolar bone, periodontal ligament, and cementum. The root is attached to bone by numerous bundles of collagenous fibers (principal fibers) that are embedded in cementum and bone (Fig. 1–9). These embedded fibers are called Sharpey's fibers. The principal fibers are named according to their location and direction of attachment (alveolar crest, horizontal, oblique, and apical). Interradicular fibers are observed on multirooted teeth.

CEMENTUM

Cementum is the calcified structure that covers the anatomic roots of teeth. It consists of a calcified matrix containing collagenous fibers. The inorganic content is approximately 45 to 50%.

PRINCIPAL FIBER GROUPS

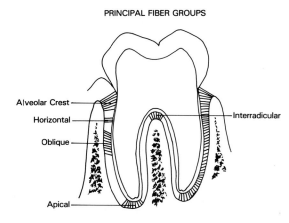

Fig. 1–9.

Cementum and Cementoid

When first formed, cementum is un-calcified and is known as cementoid. As new layers are formed, the previously formed matrix is calcified and becomes mature cementum. Microscopically, cementum can be divided into two types, cellular and acellular; functionally, however, there is no difference. The cellular cementum consists of lacunae that contain cells called cementocytes. The cells communicate with one another by means of canaliculi. The distribution of cellular and acellular cementum on the roots of teeth varies. Generally, cementum covering the coronal portion of a root is acellular, whereas that covering the apical region is cellular. Cellular cementum is also more prevalent in the bifurcation and trifurcation areas and around the apices of teeth, and is the type of cementum initially formed during wound healing.

Functions

The various functions of cementum are:

1. To anchor the tooth to the bony sockets by means of the principal fibers of the periodontal ligament.
2. To compensate, by its continuing growth, for the loss of tooth structure through wear.
3. To facilitate physiologic mesial drift of teeth.
4. To permit a continual rearrangement of the periodontal ligament.

Cementum is deposited throughout the life of a tooth. The presence of cementoid is considered a barrier to the apical migration of the junctional epithelium and to resorption of the root surface by the surrounding connective tissue.

Cementoenamel Junction

The relationships of the cementum to the enamel at the cementoenamel junction have clinical significance. There are three types of relationships, as demonstrated in Figure 1–10. In 60 to 65% of the cases, the cementum overlaps the enamel, and in 30% there is a butt joint. In 5 to 10% of patients, however, the enamel and cementum do not meet and there is exposed dentin. These patients may exhibit extreme thermal and tactile sensitivity if recession occurs. This defect also enhances the accumulation of plaque and calculus. Calculus that forms in this defect defies removal, even when visible.

Cervical Projections of Enamel

Enamel projections often extend varying distances (grades 1, 2, and 3) from the dentoenamel junction to the mid-furcal area (Figure 1–11). Their role in the spread of disease into the furcation area is unknown. Cervical projections of enamel, however, are covered by junctional epithelium rather than cementum and connective tissue fibers. An epithelial attachment is potentially weaker than a connective tissue attachment and could represent a possible pathway for early involvement of a furcation.

Palatogingival Groove

Another defect often associated with advanced periodontal destruction is the palatogingival groove (Fig. 1–12). This groove is most frequently observed on the maxillary central and lateral incisors, and

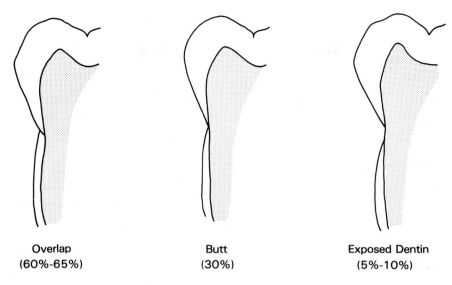

Overlap	Butt	Exposed Dentin
(60%-65%)	(30%)	(5%-10%)

Fig. 1–10.

ENAMEL PROJECTIONS

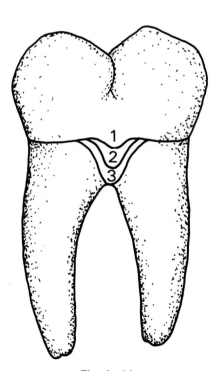

Fig. 1–11.

it often extends from the cingulum to the apex. The palatogingival groove presents a difficult, if not impossible, management problem for the patient and clinician.

ALVEOLAR PROCESS

The alveolar process is that portion of the maxilla and mandible that forms and supports the sockets (alveoli) of the teeth.

Divisions

On the basis of function and adaptation, the alveolar process can be divided into two parts.

1. *Alveolar bone proper.* A thin layer of bone that surrounds the root and gives attachment to the periodontal ligament. This bone is also known as the lamina dura or cribriform plate.
2. *Supporting alveolar bone.* The portion of the alveolar process that surrounds the alveolar bone proper and gives support to the sockets. It consists of:
   a. Compact or cortical bone found on the vestibular and oral aspects of the alveolar process.
   b. Cancellous bone (spongy bone)

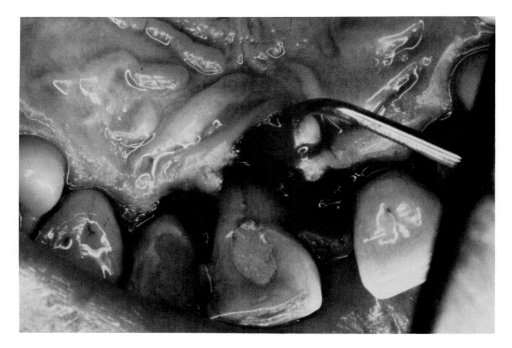

Fig. 1–12.

that lies between the alveolar bone proper and the cortical bone. Cancellous bone contains marrow that, in the adult, is mostly of the yellow or fatty type. Foci of red marrow can be found in the maxillary tuberosity and, on occasion, in the maxillary and mandibular molar and premolar areas.

Blood Supply

The vascular supply of bone is derived from intra-alveolar arteries, vessels that penetrate the cortical plates (Fig. 1–8). In circumstances under which cortical bone and alveolar bone proper are fused, as on the facial aspect of the anterior teeth, the blood supply is derived chiefly from supraperiosteal vessels.

Bundle Bone

Portions of the alveolar bone proper frequently contain "bundles" of calcified collagenous fibers from the periodontal ligament (Sharpey's fibers); these are termed bundle bone. This is not a special type of bone peculiar to tooth sockets. Bundle bone is present throughout the body, wherever tendons, ligaments, or muscles attach to bone.

Contours

The contour of the alveolar process conforms to the prominence of the roots and the position of the teeth. The height and thickness of the facial and lingual plates are affected by tooth position, root form and size, and occlusal forces. Teeth that are prominent or in labioversion often bulge through the process, resulting in either an alveolar dehiscence or an alveolar fenestration.

Teeth that are extruded, intruded, or inclined have an angular interdental crest (Fig. 1–13). Studies have shown that, in health, the alveolar crest maintains a constant distance from the cemetoenamel junction. For example, when a tooth extrudes, bone formation occurs at the al-

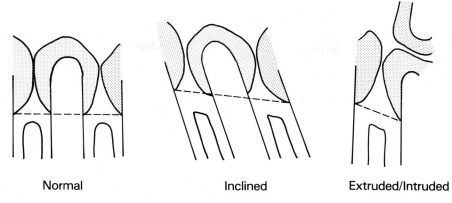

Normal   Inclined   Extruded/Intruded

Fig. 1–13.

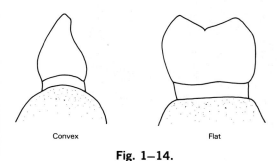

Convex   Flat

Fig. 1–14.

veolar crest, and the distance between the crest and the cementoenamel junction is maintained. This observation becomes an important factor in the radiographic interpretation of infrabony defects.

When the contour of the cementoenamel junction is broad and flat buccolingually (molars and some premolars), the contour of the alveolar process is broad and flat buccolingually (Fig. 1–14). Conversely, the buccolingual contours in the anterior region are narrow and pointed, due to the configuration of the cementoenamel junction. It has been reported that the cervical margin of the alveolar bone is often thickened in response to increased functional demands; this is called lipping, or peripheral buttressing bone formation.

Lability

Alveolar bone is the least stable of the periodontal tissues. It is extremely sensitive to both internal and external stimuli. Its contour and internal structure depend to a great extent on the stresses placed on it. For instance, in hypofunction, bone is resorbed and there is a decrease in density, with fewer and thinner trabeculae and larger medullar spaces. This state is sometimes termed disuse atrophy. Conversely, in hyperfunction, bone trabeculae are aligned in the path of tensile and compressive stresses, and there is an increase in density. When alveolar support has been weakened by periodontal disease, bone formation often occurs centrally or peripherally in an attempt to support the tooth against the occlusal forces (buttressing bone formation). When the attachment apparatus can no longer adapt to occlusal forces, the injury that occurs is termed trauma from occlusion.

Dehiscence and Fenestration

Two defects of the alveolar cortical plate, dehiscence and fenestration, have clinical and therapeutic significance. Dehiscence denotes the cleftlike absence of the alveolar cortical plate, resulting in a denuded root surface. Alveolar fenestration is a circumscribed defect in the cortical plate, exposing a facial or a lingual root surface (Fig. 1–15).

Only a very thin layer of combined cortical plate-alveolar bone proper exists over the root surfaces of teeth in labio-

ALVEOLAR DEFECTS

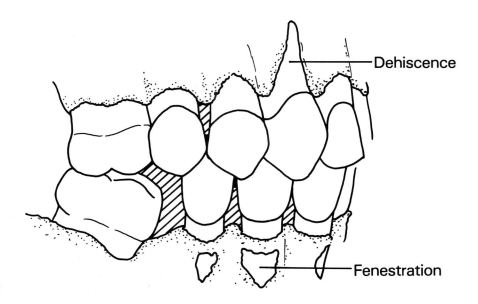

Fig. 1—15.

version, or over those with large roots. In such cases, there is only minimal, if any, interalveolar blood supply; blood supply to the bone is derived chiefly from supraperiosteal vessels. The raising of a mucoperiosteal flap and the severing of the supraperiosteal vessels may result in the loss of cortical plate, exaggeration of a dehiscence, or a fenestration becoming a dehiscence. When such defects are suspected, every effort should be made to leave connective tissue to cover the radic-

ular surface. To this end, a mucosal flap (partial-thickness flap), which preserves the supraperiosteal blood supply, is used.

A similar problem arises if bone contouring is performed over the root surfaces. According to the results of studies of wound healing, bone should rarely be removed from radicular surfaces, particularly from the cervical one-third. After osseous surgery on radicular surfaces, bone resorption continues during healing and may result in extensive osseous dehiscences.

CHAPTER 2

Etiology of Periodontal Disease

Periodontal disease may be defined as any pathologic process that affects the periodontium. The vast majority of inflammatory diseases of the periodontium result from bacterial infection. Although other factors may affect this region, the dominating causative agents of periodontal disease are microorganisms that colonize the tooth surface (bacterial plaque and their products). Figure 2–1 represents the interaction of etiologic factors that cause periodontal disease. There are a number of systemic disorders that adversely effect the periodontium (see Chapter 3), but no systemic disorder is known to cause periodontitis in the absence of bacterial plaque. In addition, there are other local factors that act in conjunction with bacterial plaque to produce chronic disease of the periodontium. Two factors that may initiate periodontal disease in the absence of bacterial plaque are malignancies and primary occlusal traumatism. The role of each factor in the initiation and progression of periodontal disease is discussed in this chapter.

TOOTH-ACCUMULATED MATERIALS (TAM)

To discuss bacterial plaque and its relationship to periodontal disease, it is necessary to define the various materials that accumulate on the tooth surface (TAM).

1. *Bacterial plaque.* A mat of densely packed, colonized, and colonizing microorganisms, that grow on and attach to the tooth. Bacterial plaque is not removed with a forceful water spray, but is readily removed by other mechanical means.
2. *Acquired pellicle.* The thin (0.1 to 0.8 μm), structureless, primarily protein film that forms on erupted teeth and can be removed by abrasives (e.g., pumice). It quickly reforms after being removed. The source of pellicle is apparently from constituents of saliva. It can form whether or not bacteria are present. Acquired pellicle will stain light pink by erythrosin, a red dye commonly used to stain bacterial plaque. Pellicle is not removed by forceful rinsing, and its role in periodontal disease is unknown.
3. *Calculus.* Calcified plaque that is usually covered by a soft layer of bacterial plaque.
4. *Food debris.* Food that is retained in the mouth. Debris, unless impacted between the teeth or within periodontal pockets, is usually removed by action of the oral musculature and saliva, or as a result of rinsing.
5. *Materia alba (literally, white matter).* A soft mixture of salivary proteins, some bacteria, many desquamated

INTERACTION OF ETIOLOGIC FACTORS

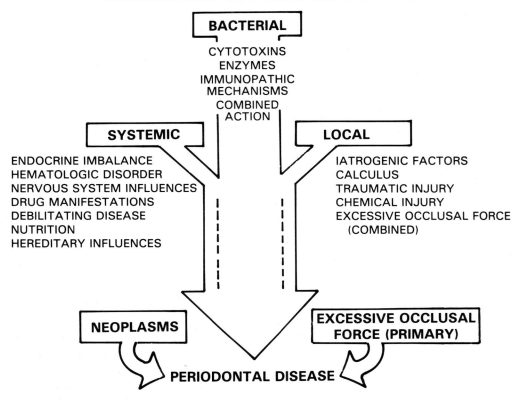

Fig. 2–1.

epithelial cells, and occasional disintegrating leukocytes. This mixture adheres loosely to the surface of the teeth, to plaque, and to gingiva, and can usually be flushed off with a forceful water spray. The toxic potential of materia alba and its role in the formation of bacterial plaque are not known.

Table 2–1 summarizes some of the differences between plaque, materia alba, and debris.

BACTERIAL FACTORS IN PERIODONTAL DISEASE

Morphology of Bacterial Plaque

Recent studies with light and electron microscopy have yielded evidence to indicate there are distinct morphologic differences between supragingival and subgingival plaque. The morphology of supragingival plaque is similar in patients with gingivitis and those with periodontitis. The bacterial cells appear to be

Table 2–1.   Some Differences between Plaque, Materia Alba, and Debris

Characteristic	Plaque	Materia Alba	Debris
Adherence	Close	Loose	None
Effect of rinsing	None	Dislodged by forceful rinsing	Dislodged readily
Structure	Definite	Amorphous	None

densely packed on the tooth surface and the deposits may be thick (0.5 mm or more). The composition of the microbial deposit includes coccoid and relatively numerous filamentous forms of bacteria. Some of the filamentous bacteria are covered with coccal organisms, which appear as "corncob" formations. Flagellated forms and spirochetes are observed apically and on the outer surface of the supragingival plaque.

Subgingival plaque in periodontitis patients is composed of an inner and an outer layer. The inner layer of tightly adherent bacteria is continuous with, but is thinner and less organized than, supragingival plaque. Outside this tightly adherent layer, and adjacent to the soft tissue of the pocket, is a loosely adherent layer of microorganisms. This layer consists of numerous spirochetes, gram-negative bacteria, and bacteria grouped into "bottle brush" or "test-tube brush" formations.

Microorganisms of Plaque

The type of microorganisms found in plaque vary among individuals and sites within the mouth, and with the age of the plaque itself. Young plaque (1 to 2 days) consists primarily of gram-positive and some gram-negative cocci and rods. These organisms normally grow on an amorphous mucopolysaccharide pellicle, less than 1 μm thick, which is attached to the enamel, cementum, or dentin.

From 2 to 4 days of growth, undisturbed plaque changes in the numbers and in the types of organisms present. The number of gram-negative cocci and rods increases and fusiform bacilli and filamentous organisms become established.

From 4 to 9 days, this ecologically complex population of microorganisms is further complicated by the presence of increasing numbers of motile bacteria, namely, spirilla and spirochetes.

It was shown recently that there are ap-

parent qualitative differences in the microbial flora associated with periodontal health and disease. Dark-field microscopy has revealed that spirochetes and motile organisms are often associated with disease whereas coccoid forms are associated with health. Studies in which plaque bacteria have been cultured show that certain gram-negative bacteria may be associated with specific types of periodontal disease. For example, *Bacteroides melaninogenicus ss intermedius* shows a strong association with minimally inflamed gingiva and advanced disease sites; *Bacteroides gingivalis* and *Fusobacterium nucleatum* are associated with adult periodontitis. *Actinobacillus actinomycetemcomitans* and strains of *Capnocytophaga* are associated with juvenile periodontitis.

Other Constituents of Plaque

Although colonized organisms are the primary constituents of plaque, additional components can be identified by phase-contrast microscopy.

1. *Epithelial cells.* These are found in almost all samples of bacterial plaque in varying stages of anatomic integrity. They may range from recently desquamated cells with discrete nuclei and clearly defined cell walls to what may be described as "ghosts" of cells swarming with bacteria.

2. *White blood cells.* Leukocytes, usually polymorphonuclear neutrophils (PMNs), may be found in varying stages of vitality in the several stages of inflammation. It is of interest that vital white cells may be found adjacent to clinically healthy gingiva. Microorganisms are often present within the cytoplasm of the granulocytes. In areas of obvious exudation and purulence, it is often difficult to find any apparently vital cells among the numerous granulocytes present.

3. *Erythrocytes.* These are readily seen

in samples taken from tooth surfaces adjacent to ulcerated gingiva.

4. *Protozoa.* Certain genera of protozoa, notably *Entamoeba* and *Trichomonas,* can often be seen in plaque taken from surfaces adjacent to acute gingivitis and from within periodontal pockets.

5. *Food particles.* Occasionally, microscopic shreds of food are seen. Those most readily recognized are muscle fibers, distinguishable by their striations.

6. *Miscellaneous components.* Nonspecific elements, such as crystalline-appearing particles (which may be fine fragments of cementum, beginning calcification, or unidentified foodstuffs) and what appear to be cell fragments, may also be found in plaque.

Mechanisms of Bacterial Action

1. *Invasion.* Bacterial invasion is not necessary for gingival inflammation to occur. All that is required is that enough bacteria (and possibly specific pathogenic bacteria) be fixed to the tooth, near the gingiva, for a sufficient length of time to challenge the tissue with their toxic products. No specific organism or group of organisms has been positively or exclusively identified as the cause of periodontal breakdown, but there appears to be a strong association of certain microorganisms with periodontal disease states. There is evidence that bacterial invasion of the connective tissue may occur.

2. *Cytotoxic agents*
   a. Endotoxins, which are lipopolysaccharide constituents of the cell wall of gram-negative bacteria, can be a direct cause of tissue necrosis, as well as an initiator of inflammation by triggering an immunologic response and activation of the complement sys-

tem. Also, endotoxins from certain oral organisms stimulate bone resorption in tissue culture.

3. *Enzymes*
   a. Collagenase depolymerizes collagen fibers and fibrils, the major formed elements in the gingiva and periodontal ligament. It is of interest that leukocytes also are known to produce collagenase and are present in large numbers in the lesions of the early stages of gingivitis.
   b. Hyaluronidase hydrolyzes hyaluronic acid, an important tissue-cementing polysaccharide, and can act as a "spreading" factor to increase tissue permeability. This enzyme is produced by microorganisms and by the host.
   c. Chondroitinase hydrolyzes chondroitin sulfate, another tissue-cementing polysaccharide.
   d. Proteases, a family of enzymes, contribute to the breakdown of noncollagenous proteins and increase capillary permeability.

4. *Immunopathologic mechanisms.* Studies have demonstrated that several plaque antigens induce inflammation in animals by stimulating the immunologic response. Both the humoral and the cell-mediated types of immune response have been observed in patients with periodontitis. The role of the immunologic response in periodontal disease is not completely understood; however, the potential to cause tissue destruction is apparent.

5. *Combined action.* It is possible that more than one mechanism may be involved in the initiation and progression of inflammatory periodontal disease. For example, it is conceivable that bacterial enzymes and/or cytotoxic substances exert a direct effect on the sulcular and subsulcular tissue, as well as initiate an

indirect immunopathologic response.

The exact mechanism of action of bacterial plaque is unknown; however, there remains little doubt that the vast majority of periodontal disease is of bacterial origin.

SYSTEMIC FACTORS AND PERIODONTAL DISEASE

Systemic factors related to periodontal disease are discussed in Chapter 3. It should be mentioned, however, that any condition that might reduce the resistance of the periodontium to toxic insult should be expected to contribute to the initiation of inflammation and to influence the rapidity and severity of the disease process.

LOCAL CONTRIBUTING FACTORS AND PERIODONTAL DISEASE

1. *Anatomic factors.* These include:
   a. Root morphology (size and shape).
   b. Position of tooth in arch.
   c. Root proximity.
2. *Iatrogenic factors.* There are a number of procedures, techniques, and materials used in dentistry that indirectly, and on occasion directly, contribute to the initiation and/or progress of periodontal disease.
   a. Operative procedures. Most injuries to the gingiva that occur during restorative dentistry procedure are of a minor nature and heal readily without loss of form or function of the periodontium. Some precautions, however, should be observed. For example, if a large portion of papilla is destroyed by careless use of a wedge during matrix stabilization, it is likely that the papilla will not regenerate to normal contour. Also, retraction cord, impression tubes, diamond stones, and temporary restorations may result in irreversible damage to the periodontium if either of the following conditions exists.
      (1) Minimal amount of attached gingiva at the operative site. The gingiva can easily become macerated and detached, with ultimate loss of all attached gingiva. Operative procedures performed under such circumstances may result in tissue loss if there is a frenum attachment at the pre-existing mucogingival junction.
      (2) The gingiva is stripped from a tooth and an overextended temporary restoration is placed, or cementing material is forced between the tooth and the detached tissue and is left in place. In either condition, epithelium will attempt to cover the detached tissue; when the temporary restoration (or cement) is finally removed, a deepened, epithelium-lined pocket will exist. The longer the materials remain interposed between tooth and soft tissue, the greater the certainty of permanent loss of the gingival attachment.
   b. Restorative materials and restorations. Except for plastics, in which excess free monomer is present, no restorative material used in dentistry today has been shown to be, in itself, capable of producing inflammation. Restorations may play a role similar to that of rough calculus if they have overhanging margins or rough surfaces. Overhanging margins and surface irregularities provide sites for plaque for-

mation and retention. The presence of overhanging margins and rough surfaces makes plaque removal difficult and provides protected areas for microorganisms to multiply and exert their toxic effect.

c. Removable partial dentures. If a prosthesis is so designed as to impinge on the soft tissue or to exert torque on the teeth, direct damage to the periodontium can occur. In the presence of bacterial plaque, these insults can result in rapid, severe destruction of periodontal structures.

d. Fixed partial dentures. In addition to the necessity for marginal excellence on abutments, the design must also be such that the patient can clean all surfaces of the restoration. This requirement demands that open interproximal embrasures and generally convex surfaces should be design elements to enhance cleanliness of the prosthesis. These principles are especially critical in pontic design. Failure to instruct patients in the methodology of cleaning fixed partial dentures is the first step toward eventual breakdown of the periodontium.

e. Exodontics. When extractions are performed so that the attachment apparatus of an adjacent tooth is damaged at or near the dentogingival junction, the damage is frequently irreversible. For example, the soft tissue and bone supporting an adjacent tooth can be destroyed if they are injudiciously used as a fulcrum for a surgical elevator. Poor flap design, as well as poor approximation and fixation of wound edges, can result in tissue contours that are conducive to plaque and food retention. Failure to remove calculus from adjacent tooth surfaces at an extraction site will negate an excellent opportunity for pocket elimination and regeneration of the attachment apparatus around the remaining teeth. This oversight indirectly enhances the progression of periodontal disease.

f. Orthodontics. Fixed appliances (bands and wires) present excellent harbors for bacterial growth and can thus contribute significantly to inflammation. Temporary extracoronal splints, whether composed of welded orthodontics bands, wire, or wire and acrylic resin, may also be included in this category.

On final analysis, it is evident that poor dentistry of all types may create sites for the accumulation of plaque, intensify its production, and prevent its mechanical removal.

3. *Calculus formation.* Calculus is calcified dental plaque. It should not be considered a direct cause of inflammation. Calculus is important in the progression of disease, however, serving as a "coral reef" within which microorganisms can multiply and release their toxic products. The rough surface of calculus makes it difficult, if not impossible, for the patient to remove associated bacterial plaque. There is ample evidence that complete removal of calculus is necessary for resolution of periodontal pockets.

4. *Traumatic.* Trauma to the periodontium can result in the loss of the attachment apparatus and can contribute to the initiation and progression of periodontal disease.

a. Toothbrush abrasion. This can completely destroy a narrow band of attached gingiva and result in extensive recession. In fact, toothbrush abrasion is one of the two most common factors associated with recession, the other being tooth position. Such abrasion also results in extensive grooving of the root surfaces, which causes cleaning problems for the patient and management problems for the dentist.

b. Factitious disease. Occasionally, patients are encountered who persistently gouge or "scratch" their gingiva with their fingernails (factitious disease). This usually results in extensive exposure of the root surface and localized inflammation. This rare entity is a difficult diagnostic problem. Whenever isolated areas of recession are noted and a thorough evaluation fails to identify the etiology of the condition, factitious disease should be considered.

c. Food impaction. This is one of the more common local factors that contribute to the initiation and progression of inflammatory periodontal disease. Open contacts, uneven marginal ridges, irregular positions of teeth, and nonphysiologic contours of teeth and restorations can result in the impaction of food on the gingiva and into the gingival sulcus. Some investigators believe that food impaction is an important factor in vertical bone loss. It is not clearly understood what pro-

duces the initial breakdown in an area of food impaction or food retention. It is speculated that the forceful wedging of food beneath the gingival tissues can produce inflammation from physical trauma, in addition to tearing of the epithelial attachment. It is just as likely, however, that the initial injury is a result of food degradation and chemical irritation. It is also possible that food impaction and retention afford an excellent breeding ground for bacteria that initiate the disease process.

5. *Chemical injury.* Indiscriminate use of aspirin tablets, strong mouthwashes, and various escharotic drugs may result in ulceration of the gingival tissue. In addition, dentists may inadvertently permit strong bleaches or salts of heavy metals, such as silver nitrate, to come in contact with the tissue. Injuries of this nature are usually transient, but may contribute to the destruction of the periodontium.

6. *Excessive occlusal force.* See Chapter 22 for a thorough discussion of this type of trauma.

Neoplasms

There are numerous benign and malignant lesions that involve the tissues of the periodontium. It is not within the scope of the *Syllabus* to discuss the various neoplasms of the periodontium, and the reader is referred to a standard text in oral pathology for this information.

CHAPTER 3

Systemic Factors Contributing to Periodontal Disease

Any systemic condition that modifies or alters the cellular metabolism may be associated with changes in the periodontal tissues. Basically, there are two ways in which systemic factors may influence periodontal tissues: 1) Acting as a predisposing factor in plaque-related periodontal disease. This is done by reducing host resistance (e.g., in diabetes) or reducing host response (e.g., immunosuppression related to chemotherapy). 2) Causing direct alteration in oral tissues. Hereditary conditions such as hypophosphatasia and hereditary gingival fibromatosis, and hypersensitivity reactions to medications and to certain foods cause tissue changes. Some of the systemic factors that can adversely affect the periodontal tissues are:

1. Aging.
2. Hereditary conditions.
3. Endocrine imbalance.
4. Hematologic disorders.
5. Nutritional status.
6. Debilitating diseases.
7. Drug manifestations.
8. Neurologic influences.

AGING

Inflammatory periodontal disease is accepted as a widespread condition that affects most people to some degree. Disease activity has been reported in children, with the prevalence increasing with age. The increased severity with aging is most likely related to the longer exposure of the periodontal tissues to the causative factors.

HEREDITARY CONDITIONS

Individuals with certain genetically determined conditions are more prone to periodontal disease because of their impaired ability to defend against local etiologic factors. Examples of these disorders include hypophosphatasia, Down's syndrome, cyclic neutropenia, and Papillon-Lefèvre syndrome. Some conditions, such as hereditary gingival fibromatosis, may be associated with changes in the periodontium without the influence of associated local precipitating factors. As yet, however, there is no conclusive evidence that heredity plays a role in the initiation and progression of inflammatory periodontal disease in man.

ENDOCRINE IMBALANCE

Diabetes Mellitus

The uncontrolled diabetic patient may be more prone to abscess formation, rapid and extensive bone loss, and intraoral fungal infections. A significant role has been identified for the polymorphonuclear leukocytes (PMN) in the periodontal response to insult. The impaired PMN function in the uncontrolled diabetic patient deserves consideration as a potential mechanism for the compromised immunologic response to inflammatory periodontal disease.

Comprehensive periodontal treatment is contraindicated for patients with uncontrolled diabetes, but not for those whose disease is under control. It is important to consult with the attending physician of all diabetic patients before initiation of periodontal therapy. The clinician must consider certain risks and limitations associated with the diabetic patient.

1. *Hypertension.* Cardiovascular disease is a common complication in individuals with diabetes. Routine blood pressure monitoring is strongly recommended.
2. *Delayed healing.* The presence of increased peripheral circulatory resistance may predispose these individuals to delayed healing.
3. *Antibiotic coverage.* Basically, the post-surgical management of the controlled diabetic patient is the same as that of a comparable nondiabetic patient. Unique circumstances of the periodontal therapy should dictate the need for antibiotic coverage.
4. *Diabetic crisis.* All surgical procedures should be performed as atraumatically as possible, preferably 2 to 3 hours after meals or after the administration of insulin.

It is important to appreciate the potential impact on the stability of a diabetic patient of any stress or infection, including chronic inflammatory periodontal disease.

Sex Hormones

Hormonal changes that occur during puberty, menstruation, or pregnancy alter the periodontal tissues to the extent that an irritant such as bacterial plaque, which initially produces a somewhat mild reaction, may change in composition and may elicit an exaggerated inflammatory response. Changes that occur in the gingiva during puberty and menstruation are hyperemia, pain, swelling, and bleeding. Changes during pregnancy may vary from a mild gingivitis to a so-called pregnancy tumor. The increased severity of inflammation will show postpartum regression, with no apparent attachment loss that is attributable to the pregnancy. A pregnancy tumor is a localized, inflammatory, hyperplastic lesion usually arising from the gingiva in the vicinity of an interdental papilla or other area of irritation or infection. Additionally, an increased severity of gingival inflammation can be seen in some women taking oral contraceptives.

Treatment of patients with hormonal imbalance usually consists of the removal of local irritating factors and instruction in plaque control. It is imperative that patients understand the serious consequences if meticulous plaque control is not carried out during periods of hormonal change. Dental procedures during pregnancy should be limited to essential therapy and in consultation with the patient's physician.

HEMATOLOGIC DISORDERS

Many patients with severe hematologic disorders, such as leukemia, are receiving chemotherapy and/or radiation, with varying degrees of success. The oral lesions of acute leukemia may consist of marked gingival hyperplasia, ulceration of the gingiva, and persistent bleeding. Patients with such oral lesions may seek dental treatment before the disease has been diagnosed. In addition, the dentist may be consulted before, during, and after chemotherapy or radiation regarding management of the oral cavity. Basically, dental treatment should be directed toward relieving pain and maintaining the best possible plaque control. The scope of dental therapy for these patients is influenced by the dental needs and the medical status of the patient.

Other forms of blood dyscrasia in which periodontal treatment should be limited are hemophilia, agranulocytosis, thrombocytopenia, and polycythemia. The various anemias may also be severe enough to impair normal cellular metabolism and thereby exert an influence on the progress and treatment of inflammatory periodontal disease.

NUTRITIONAL STATUS

Diet and Periodontal Disease

Periodontal tissues, as all body tissues, are dependent on utilization and absorption of the nutrients obtained in a balanced diet. No cause-and-effect relationship between specific nutrients and periodontal disease has been adequately shown in humans. The periodontist, however, is vitally concerned with epithelial keratinization, vascular integrity, osteogenesis, wound healing, and tissue repair—all of which are directly related to nutrition at the cellular level.

Nutritional Factors

Nutrition consists of taking in and assimilating carbohydrates, fats, proteins, vitamins, and minerals from which tissue is built and energy is liberated. It involves the processes of digestion, absorption, assimilation, and excretion. When nutrients necessary for normal functions are lacking, a nutritional deficiency occurs after a sufficient amount of time has elapsed to deplete the body's nutrient reserve. When this stage is reached, biochemical differences, functional changes, and anatomic lesions occur.

Nutritional Deficiencies

Nutritional deficiencies may be: 1) primary, resulting from insufficient food intake; or 2) secondary, resulting from impairment in the absorption, transportation, or utilization of adequate food intake. A secondary nutritional deficiency is not a result of inadequate dietary intake; rather, some factor prevents the body from utilizing or absorbing ingested food and thus causes a depletion of nutrients necessary for the tissues. Nevertheless, some dentists attempt to treat periodontal disorders by prescribing mineral supplements, various members of the vitamin B complex, or vitamin C, with little concern for the true origin of the nutritional inadequacy, or with no evidence that a deficiency exists. Indiscriminate use of doses of high-potency vitamin C to treat "bleeding gums," reduce periodontal pockets, or accelerate regeneration in wound healing has not produced the clinical results claimed by those who advocate this form of therapy.

Evaluating Nutritional Status

The clinical examination of the patient may reveal signs or symptoms suggestive of a nutritional deficiency. General weakness, fatigue, poor appetite, sore lips, sore mouth or tongue, diarrhea, or photophobia are just a few of the many signs that may indicate a need for nutritional evaluation. The first step in such an evaluation is to obtain a dietary history, listing all foodstuffs eaten for seven consecutive days. At most health centers, it is also possible to obtain a computerized analysis of the patient's dietary status. Any deficiencies noted would be considered primary nutritional deficiencies.

The second step is to discover any systemic factors that may influence the utilization and absorption of nutrients. Gastrointestinal disease, loss of appetite because of infection, food allergy, diarrhea, gallbladder disease, diabetes, thyroid disease, and adrenal dysfunction—all may contribute to a nutritional deficiency. The inactivation of vitamins such as thiamine or ascorbic acid occurs in achlorhydria; excessive amounts of oxalic acid (spinach) prevent utilization of minerals by the body; polyuria associated with diabetes or fever affects the nitrogen retention of the tissues as well as the water balance of the body; sprue, ulcerative colitis, dysentery, and other diseases that interfere with fat absorption, inhibit the absorption of the fat-soluble vitamins A, D, E, and K. These factors may be considered secondary if an adequate diet has been maintained.

In the presence of serious systemic disease, the dentist should refer the patient to a physician for dietary counseling and therapy. In general, whenever nutritional inadequacies are suspected, the patient's physician should be consulted.

DEBILITATING DISEASES

Diseases that debilitate the patient may also have effects on the periodontal tissues. The response to irritants, healing, and regenerative capacities of the periodontal tissues may be altered by some types of debilitating disease, such as lupus erythematosus, pemphigus, and pemphigoid. The more significant effect of debilitating disease is related to the limitation of many of these patients to perform adequate plaque removal. Patients with debilitating disease, such as arthritis and scleroderma, present special challenges to the clinician in the treatment and the establishment of an adequate plaque-control program.

DRUG MANIFESTATIONS

Reactions to certain drugs produce changes in the gingival tissue that can manifest as an enlargement, ulceration, or diffuse tissue involvement.

1. *Heavy metals.* Ingestion of metals such as bismuth, lead, and mercury produces a linear pigmentation in the gingiva.
2. *Phenytoin.* This drug, used in the treatment of epilepsy, is frequently associated with marked gingival hyperplasia (dilantin hyperplasia). Hyperplastic changes appear first in the interdental papilla; in advanced cases the teeth may be completely covered.
3. *Food and medication.* The ingestion of some foods and medications can produce a hypersensitivity reaction in the oral tissues, such as in the lesions of allergic gingivostomatitis, plasma cell gingivitis, and erythema multiforme.
4. *Chemotherapy agents.* These may:
   a. Lower the patient's ability to cope with infections and impair healing, as related to the systemic administration of cortisone and other adrenal corticosteroids.
   b. Cause a direct effect on oral tissues, resulting in tissue breakdown with ulcerations and discomfort.

NEUROLOGIC INFLUENCES

Autonomic nervous system influences may cause local alterations in blood supply and thereby impair tissue nutrition. Autonomic influences may also affect the periodontium by eliciting changes in salivary flow.

Psychologic problems may cause occlusal neuroses, interfere with oral hygiene and diet, or initiate undesirable oral habits (factitious gingival abrasion). The high prevalence of periodontal disease in patients with mental disorders is probably related to the inadequate plaque control generally associated with these patients.

CHAPTER 4

Plaque-Related Periodontal Disease: Pathogenesis and Immune Response

The pathogenesis of a disease refers to the biologic and histologic events that occur in the tissues during the process of conversion from a healthy state to a diseased state. Understanding the pathogenesis of periodontal disease will allow the clinician to make rational decisions regarding the most predictable methods to prevent and/or treat this widespread disease.

TYPES OF PLAQUE-RELATED PERIODONTAL DISEASE

Gingivitis

Gingivitis is inflammation of the gingiva. There is no loss of attachment associated with this condition. The clinical findings may consist of redness of the gingival margin, varying degrees of swelling, bleeding on gentle probing, and alterations in physiologic gingival architecture. Pain is not a common finding in gingivitis. The clinical and histologic features are summarized in Table 4–1.

Periodontitis

Periodontitis is inflammation of the periodontium characterized by apical migration of the junctional epithelium with associated loss of attachment and crestal alveolar bone. The clinical findings include increased probing depth, bleeding on probing (in active disease states), and alteration of physiologic contour. Redness and swelling of the gingiva may also be present. Pain is not a common clinical finding.

Pocket Formation

A pocket is a gingival sulcus pathologically deepened by periodontal disease. It is bordered by the tooth on one side, by ulcerated epithelium on the other, and has the junctional epithelium at its base. Deepening of the sulcus can occur in three ways: 1) by movement of the free gingival margin coronally, as observed in gingivitis; 2) by movement of the junctional epithelium apically, with separation of the coronal portion from the tooth; and 3) by a combination of items 1) and 2) (Fig. 4–1).

Classification of Pockets

Pockets may be classified as follows (Fig. 4–2):

1. *Gingival pocket (pseudo-pocket).* Deepening of the gingival sulcus as a result of an increase in the size of the gingiva. There is no apical migration of the junctional epithelium or loss of crestal bone (Fig. 4–2*a*).

Table 4–1. Clinical and Histologic Features of Gingivitis

Clinical Change	Underlying Histologic Changes
Gingival bleeding	Ulceration of sulcular epithelium, with engorged capillaries extending near surface
Redness	Hyperemia, with dilatation and engorgement of capillaries
Swelling, puffiness	Infiltration of connective tissues by fluid and cells of inflammatory exudate
Loss of gingival tone	Inflammation, with destruction of gingival fiber apparatus
Loss of stippling	Edema underlying connective tissue
Firm, leathery consistency	Fibrosis associated with long-standing chronic inflammation
Gingival pocket	Inflammation, with ulceration of sulcular epithelium and gingival enlargement

POCKET FORMATION

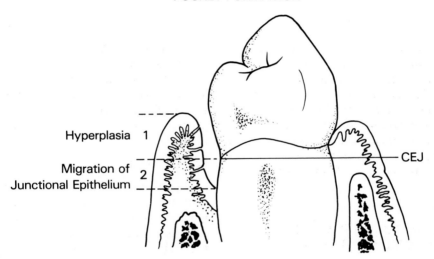

Fig. 4–1.

CLASSIFICATION OF POCKETS

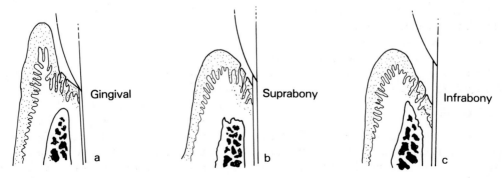

Fig. 4–2.

2. *Suprabony pocket.* Deepening of the gingival sulcus—with destruction of the adjacent gingival fibers, periodontal ligament, and alveolar bone—associated with apical migration of the junctional epithelium. The bottom of the pocket and the junctional epithelium are coronal to the crest of the alveolar bone (Fig. 4–2b).

3. *Infrabony pocket.* Deepening of the gingival sulcus to a level at which the bottom of the pocket and the junctional epithelium are apical to the crest of the alveolar bone (Fig. 4–2c) One, two, or three osseous walls, or various combinations thereof, may remain, depending on the amount and pattern of bone loss (see Chapter 16 for classification of osseous defects).

Horizontal and Vertical Bone Loss

Horizontal bone loss refers to an overall reduction in height of the alveolar crest in which the crestal bone is at right angles to the root surface. Vertical bone loss refers to loss of bone at an acute angle to the root surface. Another term for vertical bone loss is angular bone loss. Suprabony pockets are associated with horizontal bone loss (Fig. 4–2b); infrabony pockets are associated with vertical bone loss (Fig. 4–2c).

Etiology of the Infrabony Pocket

Both suprabony and infrabony pockets are the result of plaque infection; however, there is some difference of opinion as to the factors that influence the formation of the infrabony pocket. Most agree that vertical bone loss and subsequent infrabony pocket formation can occur whenever there is direct extension of inflammation into the periodontal ligament, in the presence of a sufficient thickness of bone. The controversy arises as to what factors alter the pathway of inflammation from crestal bone to the

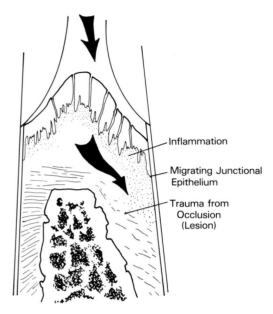

PERIODONTAL TRAUMATISM

Inflammation

Migrating Junctional Epithelium

Trauma from Occlusion (Lesion)

Fig. 4–3.

periodontal ligament space. The etiologic mechanisms that have been proposed are as follows.

1. Large vessels that exit on one side of the alveolus may affect formation of an infrabony pocket.

2. The forceful wedging of food into the interproximal region may result in unilateral destruction of the attachment apparatus and downgrowth of the epithelial attachment.

3. Periodontal traumatism may produce crestal damage of the periodontal ligament (trauma from occlusion) that, in the presence of existing inflammation, can result in the migration of the junctional epithelium into the area of destruction (Fig. 4–3) (see Chapter 22).

Juvenile Periodontitis (Periodontosis)

Localized juvenile periodontitis (LJP) is a disease that primarily affects a small percentage of adolescents. The classic appearance of LJP is characterized by severe bone loss about the permanent first molars and permanent incisor teeth, sparse plaque formation (relative absence of local factors), and minimal gingival inflammation. The disease has a predilection for females with a 3:1 female-to-male ratio. Certain gram-negative anaerobes show a strong relationship to this condition. One of the microorganisms, *Actinobacillus actinomycetemcomitans,* strain Y4, produces substances that could play a prominent role in the extensive tissue destruction seen in LJP. These substances include: a leukotoxin that is toxic to leukocytes, collagenase, endotoxin, and a fibroblast inhibitory factor. There is also a form of the disease called generalized juvenile periodontitis, which involves most of the dentition.

The treatment regimen should include initiation of an effective plaque control program, thorough root detoxification, and flap surgery to remove granulomatous tissue and to gain access to the root surface. In addition, there is evidence that 1 g of tetracycline administered daily, in four equally divided doses, over a 10- to 21-day period will improve the clinical result.

PATHOGENESIS OF PLAQUE-RELATED PERIODONTAL DISEASE

Plaque-related periodontal disease is characterized by inflammation. The inflammatory process is activated to limit the spread of the disease process. In addition to its beneficial effects, however, the inflammatory process also has a destructive component. The objective of treatment is to enhance the beneficial aspects of inflammation and to limit or control the destructive potential.

The inflammatory response in plaque-related periodontal disease can be initiated by a variety of factors. There is evidence that a number of the lytic enzymes produced by bacteria can cause direct tissue destruction in the periodontium.

Other bacterial products (e.g., endotoxin) may activate the complement system, which results in the formation of biologically active proteins that cause, inter alia, an increase in vascular permeability with migration of inflammatory cells from the vascular channels, the chemotactic response, and phagocytosis. The end result of complement activation is cell lysis.

The immunologic response appears to play a significant role in the initiation, and probably the perpetuation, of the inflammatory response. The bacteria in plaque contain a multitude of antigens. The antigens can stimulate the B and T lymphocytes of the gingival connective tissues to proliferate, and contribute to both the humoral and cell-mediated immune response, respectively. To support this concept, there is evidence that patients with plaque-related periodontal disease have circulating antibodies to plaque antigens. It also has been shown that cultures of peripheral lymphocytes from patients with plaque-related periodontal disease show a greater cell-mediated immune response to plaque-derived antigens than peripheral lymphocytes from periodontally healthy patients.

Histopathology

The histologic picture of developing plaque-related periodontal disease has been divided into four stages (the model proposed by Page and Schroeder).

The Initial Lesion

The first microscopically observable tissue changes occur after 2 to 4 days of plaque accumulation. There are small accumulations of polymorphonuclear neutrophils (PMNs) and mononuclear cells subjacent to the junctional epithelium. A decrease of perivascular collagen occurs in this area as well as a decrease of some of the collagen supporting the coronal portion of the junctional epithelium. Gingival fluid can be detected clinically in the gingival sulcus; no more than 5 to 10%

of the gingival connective tissue is involved during this stage.

The Early Lesion

The early lesion occurs after 4 to 7 days of plaque accumulation. The changes observed in the initial lesion persist and are more severe at this stage. Numerous small and medium-sized lymphocytes accumulate immediately below the junctional epithelium. These cells are the predominant inflammatory cells. The junctional and oral sulcular epithelium begin to form rete pegs. Numerous injured fibroblasts are observed in close association with lymphoid cells. The collagen content is reduced about 70% in the areas of inflammation.

The Established Lesion

The established lesion is observed after 2 to 3 weeks of plaque accumulation. The destructive tissue changes noted in the first two stages persist. The plasma cell is now the predominant inflammatory cell type. These cells produce immunoglobulins, primarily of the IgG class. The junctional and oral sulcular epithelium continue to proliferate and may now be considered pocket epithelium. This epithelium varies in thickness and shows areas of ulceration. The inflammatory cells accumulate along vascular channels and between collagen fibers deep in the lesion. The collagen loss persists at the site of active disease, but areas distant from the lesion show foci of collagen formation. The periodontal ligament and alveolar bone show no change at this stage. Clinical manifestations of the disease can now be observed.

The Advanced Lesion

A varying amount of time elapses before the advanced lesion occurs. There are many cases in which the advanced lesion never appears. The area of the lesion enlarges. Strands of pocket epithelium penetrate deep into the connective tissue.

There is extensive destruction of the collagen fiber bundles and of the gingiva; however, the transseptal fibers continually regenerate as the lesion moves apically. The plasma cell continues to be the predominant cell type. Many of these cells appear injured, and can be observed deep within the tissue. Crestal alveolar bone resorption occurs, especially in the area of the vascular channels.

Disease Progression

The initial, early, and established lesions represent varying severities of gingivitis. The advanced lesion can be considered periodontitis. All the events in one stage in the life cycle of plaque-related periodontal disease need not be completed before another stage begins. The stages are a continuum of the disease process, with considerable overlap between stages. Periodontitis must be preceded by gingivitis; however, all untreated gingivitis does not necessarily proceed to periodontitis.

Progression of periodontal disease is now considered a cyclic process. There appear to be extended periods of quiescence with short episodes of disease activity. The attachment loss that occurs during these bursts of disease activity varies from minor loss to relatively extensive tissue loss.

Spread of Inflammation

Periodontitis usually develops as a sequel to persistent chronic gingivitis. Interdentally, inflammation and bacterial products spread from the gingiva to the alveolar process along the neurovascular bundle of the interdental canal at the crest of the septum (Fig. 4–4a1). Inflammation spreads along the course of the vascular channels because the loose connective tissue surrounding the neurovascular bundles offers less resistance than the dense fibers of the periodontal ligament. The point at which inflammation enters the bone depends on the location of the ves-

SPREAD OF INFLAMMATION

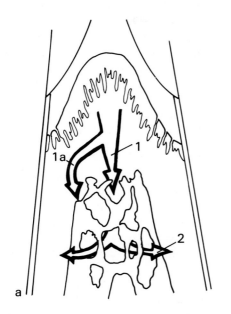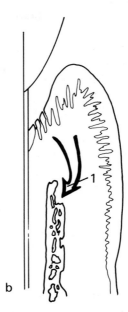

Fig. 4—4.

sels. In some instances, large vessels exit at one side of the alveolar crest, permitting direct spread of inflammation into the marginal portion of the periodontal ligament (Fig. 4–4a and *1a*). After reaching the marrow spaces, the destructive process extends laterally into the periodontal ligament via the intra-alveolar opening (Fig. 4–4a2). On the facial and lingual surfaces, the destructive process speeds along the supraperiosteal vessels and penetrates the marrow space via the channels in the outer cortex (Fig. 4–4b1).

Extension of the chronic inflammatory process into the alveolar bone is marked by infiltration of the marrow by leukocytes, new blood vessels, and proliferation of fibroblasts. There is marked osteoclas-

Table 4–2.   Clinical Findings and Histologic Features of Periodontitis

Clinical Finding	Histologic Feature
Bleeding and pain on probing	Ulceration of sulcular epithelium
Blue-red discoloration of gingiva	Circulatory stagnation of chronic inflammation
Smooth, shiny gingival surface with loss of stippling	Atrophy of the epithelium and edema
Flaccidity of gingiva	Destruction of the gingival fiber apparatus
Exposed root surfaces	Result of long-standing chronic inflammation, with progressive apical movement of junctional epithelium and gingival margin, and corresponding loss of alveolar process
Occasionally pink, firm, heavily stippled gingiva with deep pocket formation	Reparative phase of inflammation predominating over the exudative and degenerative phase; pocket wall, however, presents degenerative changes and ulceration
Suppuration	Ulceration of epithelium, not indicative of severity of disease process or depth of pocket

tic activity. Progressive extension is accompanied by destruction of the trabeculae and subsequent reduction in the height of the alveolar bone. This destruction is not a continuous process; it is accompanied by osteoblastic activity and new bone formation, even in the presence of inflammation. Likewise, there is constant reformation of the transseptal fibers as the attachment apparatus is destroyed. Alveolar bone loss does not occur until the physiologic equilibrium of bone is disturbed to the point that resorption exceeds formation. The resistance to disease of the individual plays an important role in governing the rate at which bone loss progresses in untreated periodontal disease.

Clinical Findings Correlated with Histologic Features

The significance of the clinical findings in periodontitis are more easily understood if they can be correlated with the histologic features of the disease (Table 4–2).

CHAPTER 5

Diagnosis, Prognosis, and Treatment Planning

The successful management of periodontal disease depends on the systematic conversion of examination data into a comprehensive, written treatment plan. Diagnosis, prognosis, and treatment planning are certainly three of the most important services that we perform in dentistry. To be a good diagnostician, one must gather all the facts, sort them and then assimilate them into a step-by-step road map or treatment plan. The meticulous manner in which the clinician approaches the fact-gathering appointment(s) will determine the success or failure of case management. This chapter is designed to serve as a guide for the gathering of information, and to discuss its use in the formation of a prognosis and treatment plan.

DIAGNOSIS

Periodontal Chart

The practitioner's approach to periodontal diseases will be more productive and less frustrating if information is recorded on a form that serves as a fact-gathering guide, allows brief shorthand notations, and provides space in which to formulate the treatment plan.

The basic means of gathering data that precede periodontal therapy may be considered as a series of surveys. As these surveys are completed, it may be helpful to estimate the comparative influence of each survey area on the patient's condition. The survey areas are:

1. Health survey.
2. General dental survey.
3. Periodontal survey.
4. Occlusal survey.
5. Radiographic survey.
6. Deposits survey.

Stated simply, virtually all periodontal disease is a struggle between the patient's resistance factors and dentobacterial plaque. Every single factor surveyed simply modifies the influence of either the disease agent or the host resistance.

Health Survey

The health survey includes a medical and a dental history.

Medical History

A medical history should be obtained first by a written questionnaire. Once the written questionnaire is complete, it should be reviewed with the patient so a thorough explanation of any areas of concern may be provided. This is the appropriate time to refer patients for a medical consultation if any condition exists that might affect the progression of the periodontal disease and/or the management of the patient.

A medical history is vital for three major reasons:

1. To detect oral manifestations of certain systemic conditions. These may include leukemia, diabetes mellitus, hormonal disturbance, etc. An alert diagnostician, in addition to ensuring good management for his patient, may detect conditions having important health implications.

2. To ascertain systemic conditions, such as pregnancy, diabetes mellitus, blood dyscrasias, nutritional deficiencies, and hypertensive cardiovascular diseases that may alter the response of the host to the bacterial insult.

3. To determine certain systemic conditions that require modification of both primary and supportive periodontal therapy. These include allergic conditions, rheumatic fever syndrome, diabetes mellitus, endocrine disorders, cardiovascular diseases and valvular prostheses, drug therapy (endocrine, corticosteroid, anticoagulant), and psychologic problems.

An example of the importance of the medical history is in the treatment of patients with valvular damage or valvular prostheses. It is imperative that the therapist immediately recognize patients in this clinical condition. Any probing or manipulation of the gingival tissue (periodontal examination, scaling, curettage, root canal treatment, extractions, periodontal surgery, etc.) that causes bleeding results in bacteremia, which could result in subacute bacterial endocarditis.

Patients who have cardiovascular problems should be managed in coordination with a physician, preferably a cardiologist. A written consultation should be obtained and retained as a permanent part of the patient's record. Occasionally, patients who claim a history of rheumatic fever are reported by the cardiologist to be free from valvular damage or associated sequelae, thereby negating the need for antibiotic coverage. It is extremely important, however, that all patients with a history of rheumatic fever be carefully evaluated by a physician before any dental treatment is rendered. Consultation in writing—not by telephone—is preferred.

The patient at risk for bacterial endocarditis should be given antibiotic coverage. The American Medical Association, the American Heart Association, and the American Dental Association have endorsed the following regimens:

Antibiotic prophylaxis is recommended with all dental procedures (including routine professional cleaning) likely to cause gingival bleeding. Because alpha-hemolytic (viridans) streptococci are most commonly implicated in endocarditis after dental procedures, prophylaxis should be specifically directed against these organisms.

Persons at risk for bacterial endocarditis are those with prosthetic cardiac valves (including biosynthetic ones), most congenital heart malformations, surgically constructed systemic pulmonary shunts, rheumatic and other acquired valvular dysfunctions, idiopathic hypertrophic subaortic stenosis (IHSS), a previous history of bacterial endocarditis, and mitrovalve prolapse with insufficiency.

Prophylaxis Recommendations for Dental Procedures and Surgery of Upper Respiratory Tract

1. Standard Regimen

    Oral penicillin. For adults and children over 60 pounds: Penicillin V 2.0 g 1 hour before the procedure and then 1.0 g 6 hours later.

    For patients unable to take *oral* antibiotics before a procedure,

2,000,000 units of aqueous penicillin G (50,000 U/kg for children) intraveniously (IV) or intramuscularly (IM) 30 to 60 minutes before the procedure and 1,000,000 units (25,000 U/kg for children) 6 hours later may be substituted.

2. For patients with prosthetic valves and others with the highest risk of endocarditis (e.g., those with prosthetic heart valves or surgically constructed systemic-pulmonary shunts), the committee favors *parenteral* ampicillin and gentamycin.

   Ampicillin 1.0 to 2.0 g (50 mg/kg for children) plus gentamycin 1.5 mg/kg (2.0 mg/kg for children) both IM or IV one-half hour before the procedure, followed by 1 g oral penicillin V (500 mg for children under 60 pounds) 6 hours later. Alternatively, the parenteral regimen should be repeated once 8 hours later. (Children's antibiotic dosage should not exceed the maximum adult dosage.)

3. Standard regimen for patients *allergic to penicillin.*

   Oral erythromycin. Erythromycin 1.0 g (20 mg/kg for children) 1 hour before the procedure, then 500 mg (10 mg/kg for children) 6 hours later. (Children's antibiotic dosage should not exceed the maximum adult dosage.)

   For patients unable to tolerate oral erythromycin, changing to a different erythromycin preparation may be beneficial. For those who cannot tolerate either penicillin or erythromycin, an oral cephalosporin (1.0 g 1 hour before the procedure plus 500 mg 6 hours later) may be useful, but data are lacking to allow specific recommendations for this regimen. Tetracyclines *cannot* be recommended for this purpose.

4. Regimen for *high risk* patients *allergic to penicillin* (high risk patients again are those with prosthetic heart valves, surgically constructed pulmonary shunts, etc.).

   Vancomycin IV. Vancomycin 1 g (20 mg/kg for children), IV slowly over 1 hour starting 1 hour before the procedure. (Children's antibiotic dosage should not exceed the maximum adult dosage.) Because of the long half-life of vancomycin, a repeat dose should not be necessary.

A greater and more detailed explanation of the above guidelines can be found in a special report in the Journal of the American Dental Association, *110*(1):98–100, 1985.

Patients with cardiovascular problems are only one example of the importance of a thorough medical history. The often repeated phrase "never treat a stranger" is good advice.

Dental History

Before the intraoral examination, a complete dental history should be obtained. By doing so, the practitioner is afforded the opportunity to assay the patient's attitude, establish rapport, and learn of past dental disease and response to treatment. It is also important to determine what methods of tooth cleansing the patient is presently using, and his general dental I.Q.

General Dental Survey

The overall impression gained by this survey will begin to establish the magnitude of the problem. The following points should be observed and noted.

1. *Soft tissue survey.* This is the oral cancer search. Other lesions must be noted also, but few have consequences as severe, especially if not detected early or if completely overlooked.
2. *Positioning.* Arch alignment, morphologic malocclusion, and migration of teeth.
3. *Caries.* Location, type, and extent.

4. *Restorative dentistry.* Adequacy of restorations and prostheses. These must be viewed in relation to plaque retention, prevention of plaque removal, traumatogenic occlusion, and excessive leverage from torquing forces.
5. *Habits.* Examples include smoking, tongue-thrusting, bruxism, and clenching.
6. *Pulpal status of teeth with advanced bone loss* (particularly when associated with teeth that have deep restorations and/or furcation involvement). The relationships between pulpal status and periodontal disease have become increasingly important and may alter treatment planning.
7. *Mobility of teeth.* This is a critical diagnostic and prognostic consideration. Some mobility is normal and may vary during the day, according to diet and stress. Pathologic mobility has several principal causes:
   a. Gingival and periodontal inflammation.
   b. Parafunctional occlusal habits.
   c. Occlusal prematurities.
   d. Loss of supporting bone.
   e. Traumatic torquing forces applied to clasped teeth by removable partial dentures.
   f. Periodontal therapy, endodontic therapy, and trauma may cause transient mobility.

Tooth movement is measured by applying force buccolingually between two dental instrument handles. Mobility is usually graded as 1, 2, or 3 (Fig. 5–1). Grade 1 represents the first distinguishable sign of movement greater than normal; Grade 2 is recorded if there is a total movement of about 1 mm; Grade 3 is recorded if the tooth moves more than 1 mm in any direction and/or is depressible. Reduction or control of pathologic tooth mobility may be achieved through re-

GRADES OF MOBILITY

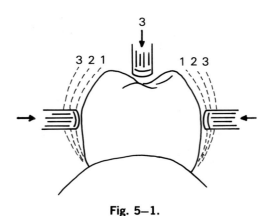

Fig. 5–1.

moval or modification of the causative factors.

Periodontal Survey

This survey is a critical part of the diagnostic process. A calibrated periodontal probe, a cowhorn or pigtail explorer, a front reflective surface examining mirror, adequate light, palpation, and air blast must all be employed to supplement visual examination of the periodontal tissues. Figures 5–2 demonstrates how information obtained from a periodontal survey may be recorded.
1. *Gingival color, form, and consistency.* These should be observed and recorded.
2. *Bleeding and purulent exudation.* These are clinical indicators of disease activity and should be noted. Exudation may be spontaneous or may be evident only on probing or palpation. Bleeding and suppuration are not indicators of the severity of the disease, but may signify ulceration of the epithelial wall of the pocket, with a corresponding reaction of the body to infection.
3. *Pocket depth.* Measurement is taken from the gingival margin on all teeth with the aid of a calibrated probe. The instrument is held as close to

the tooth surface as possible and is gently inserted into the sulcus or pocket until resistance is met. Any bleeding or suppuration is recorded. The probe is walked along the tooth surface, keeping it parallel to the long axis of the tooth. Three measurements are recorded on both the facial and lingual surfaces: distal, midfacial/midlingual, and mesial (Fig. 5–3) When there is heavy calculus formation, it is often impossible to measure pocket depth accurately, because calculus will impede the insertion of the probe. It may then be necessary to perform a gross debridement before pocket measurement.

4. *Relationship of gingival margin to cementoenamel junction (recession).* This information is recorded as a continuous line on a chart. If this step is neglected, pocket measurements are meaningless. A 3-mm pocket, for example, on a tooth with 5 mm of gingival recession would signify greater destruction of the attachment apparatus than a 5-mm pocket on a tooth with hyperplastic gingiva (Fig. 5–4).

5. *General width of keratinized gingiva, relationship of pocket depth to mucogingival junction, and influence of various frenal and muscle attachments on gingival margin.* These should be observed and recorded.

6. *Pathologic invasion of furcation areas.* Careful probing with a curved explorer will make this determination. The complicated anatomy of these regions presents diagnostic and therapeutic challenges. Furcations and classification are discussed in Chapter 18.

Occlusal Survey

Because occlusion may influence the progress and severity of periodontal disease, the occlusal status of every patient should be evaluated. An occlusal survey will enable the therapist to gauge the relative importance of occlusion in each individual case and to determine whether occlusal adjustment is indicated.

Analysis of the Occlusion

Certain information must be obtained before a final evaluation of the role of occlusion can be made.

Clinical Evaluation. The clinician must:

1. Determine parafunctional habits (e.g., bruxing, clenching, doodling, and fingernail biting).
   [The following information must be obtained with the patient in an upright position.]

2. Identify the initial tooth contact in centric relation. This is a reference point from which the occlusion can be adjusted. To find the initial contact in centric relation, place gentle pressure against the center of the mandible and guide the mandible posteriorly (Fig. 5–5). Record the first contact in centric relation (first centric prematurity) by tapping the teeth into occlusal indicator wax or articulating ribbon.

3. Determine the anterior slide of the mandible. Have the patient slowly close the teeth completely from the initial contact in centric relation; observe anterior or lateral movement of the mandible. Also note any facial movement of the maxillary anterior teeth as the jaw closes from centric relation to functional (habitual) occlusion.

4. Determine prematurities in functional occlusion. This is the position in which most tooth contacts occur (Fig. 5–6).

5. Determine working contacts. Working contacts occur when the mandible is moved laterally from functional occlusion with the teeth in contact. The patient is asked to glide the mandible right and left from the

Periodontics Chart

1. Date of Examination: 7/31/84
   Date of Treatment Completed: _____

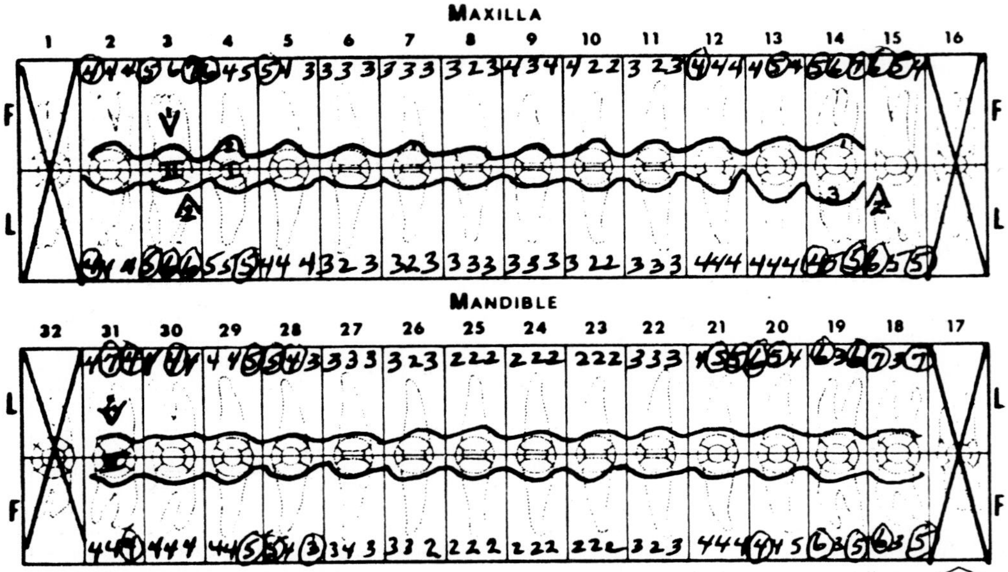

MAXILLA

1   2   3   4   5   6   7   8   9   10   11   12   13   14   15   16

MANDIBLE

32   31   30   29   28   27   26   25   24   23   22   21   20   19   18   17

KEY FOR CHARTING Mobility I. II. III   Food Impaction ↓   Furca Involvement 1, 2, 3
Missing Teeth X   To be Extracted = TE   or Poor Contact ↓   Overhang JL

10. Periodontal Case Types:

Case Type I — Gingivitis — Shallow pockets — No bone loss
Case Type I-A — Gingivitis with complicating factors
Case Type II — Early periodontitis (mod pockets, minor bone loss)
Case Type II-A — Early periodontitis with complicating factors
Case Type III — Moderate periodontitis
Case Type III-A — Moderate periodontitis with complicating factors
Case Type IV — Advanced periodontitis
Case Type IV-A — Advanced periodontitis with complicating factors
Case Type V — Special case requiring specific single procedure
Case Type V-A — Special case requiring narrative report

11. Prognosis: Excellent – Good – Fair – Poor – Hopeless

12. Treatment Plan:

1. _____   8. _____
2. _____   9. _____
3. _____   10. _____
4. _____   11. _____
5. _____   12. _____
6. _____   13. _____
7. _____   14. _____

Treatment Time: _____ visits over _____ weeks/mos
Approved by: _____
                    Instructors Signature

13. Fee: _____

15. Plaque Index:

Date	7/31/84				
Operator	J				
Index	108/128				

14. Pre-Op Photos: Date: 7/31/84
Ant. ✓, Lft ✓, Rt ✓, Ling ✓, Palatal ✓

Fig. 5–2.

2. Radiographic Interpretation: _generalized horizontal bone loss except_ _vertical bone loss notes mesial #3, Double mesial #18_

3. Study Cast Analysis: _____

4. Case History (chief complaint, medical, and dental history): _Toothache, bleeding_ _gums and loose teeth_

5. Mobility Patterns: _Class I #4 ; Class II #3 + #1_

6. Prosthesis Evaluation: _N.A._

7. Gingival Tissues (color, tone, form, contour, recession): _Red, inflamed, edematous_ _recession noted # 4, 7, 14_

8. Occlusal Evaluation: _Canthia prematurity # 2/31_

9. Review of Findings: _____

15. Initial Plaque Control Instructions and Aids Prescribed: _Sulcular Cleansing,_ _Floss, Perio aid_

16. Recall and Maintenance Prescribed: _____

17. Date	Treatment

Fig. 5–2. *Continued*

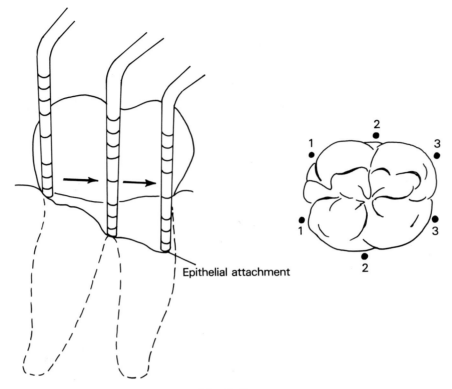

Epithelial attachment

Fig. 5—3.

RECESSION HYPERPLASIA

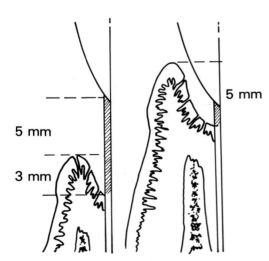

Fig. 5—4.

functional position. Working contacts are best recorded with ribbon.

6. Determine balancing (nonworking) contacts. When the mandible is moved to the right (right working), posterior teeth may contact on the left. These contacts are called balancing (nonworking) contacts. They are located by placing ribbon on the nonworking side and having the patient move the mandible into working position. Look for long, streaked markings on the teeth.

7. Determine contacts in protrusive position. Have the patient bite on the anterior teeth in tip-to-tip relation. Also note any posterior teeth that may contact in this position.

8. Determine protrusive excursion. Place the ribbon between the upper and lower anterior teeth. Have the patient close in functional position

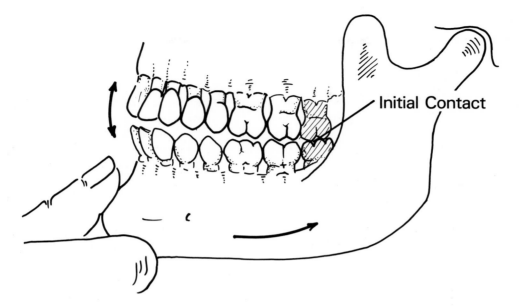

Fig. 5–5.

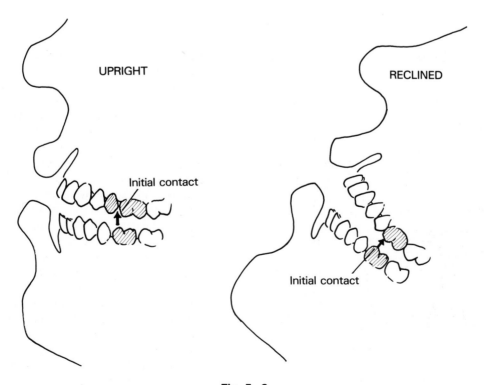

Fig. 5–6.

and then protrude the mandible until the teeth reach protrusive position.

9. Check movement of teeth during chewing (fremitus). Place the ball of the index finger on the teeth one at a time and determine if the tooth moves as the patient glides the mandible into working or protrusive position.

10. Determine tooth/tooth relationships: open contacts, irregular contacts, food impaction sites, rough incisal/occlusal surfaces. These may often be detected on the study casts.

Evaluation of Study Casts. The following information may be obtained from study casts:

1. Plunger cusps.
2. Wear facets.
3. Malposed teeth.
4. Abnormal marginal ridge relationship.
5. Condition of existing restorations (contour buccolingual dimension).
6. First molar relationship (Angle's classification).
7. Overbite (vertical overlap of teeth).
8. Overjet (horizontal overlap of teeth).

Periodontal Trauma from Occlusion

Once the occlusal survey is complete, the clinician must relate the data to the existence or nonexistence of trauma from occlusion. The following outline of signs and symptoms will serve as a guide in diagnosis.

Clinical Signs. These include:

1. Passive mobility of teeth.
2. Fremitus.
3. Migration of teeth, especially "fanning" of anterior teeth.
4. Unusual wear patterns of teeth (facets).
5. Hypertonicity of masticatory muscles.
6. Periodontal abscess formation, especially in deep infrabony defects and furcas.

Symptoms. Trauma from occlusion is often asymptomatic, but the following symptoms may be indicative of this condition:

1. Soreness on percussion and in function. This is often associated with new restorations and has a short-term history. In chronic periodontal traumatism, pain may be more vague and generalized.
2. Pain and spasm in muscles of mastication.
3. Food impaction due to forceful wedging by opposing teeth.
4. Temporomandibular joint or myofascial pain/dysfunction syndrome.
5. "Looseness of teeth," vague "itching," and tendency to grind or initiate parafunction on certain teeth.
6. Thermal hypersensitivity of teeth.

Radiographic Signs. Radiography permits identification of characteristic evidence of trauma from occlusion.

1. Alterations in the lamina dura:
   a. Uneven thickening may be associated with tensional forces, but is unreliable.
   b. Severe occlusal force may cause a complete loss.
2. Alteration in the periodontal ligament space. Widening may mean increased function or periodontal traumatism. The widening may be compensatory, especially if the lamina dura is thickened and intact.
3. Root resorption. This may be due to excessive force in orthodontics, bruxism, or reconstruction therapy.
4. Hypercementosis. This may be a compensatory phenomenon to increase resistance to occlusal forces.
5. Osteosclerosis. Signs of this condition may occasionally be observed.
6. Angular bone loss and bone loss in furcation areas. These have been suggested in association with excessive occlusal force.

7. Root fracture.

Microscopic Changes. Various functional conditions, including trauma from occlusion, may produce changes within the periodontium that can be observed microscopically.

1. Changes that may result from nonfunction:
   a. Widened bone marrow spaces.
   b. Thin and disoriented trabeculae.
   c. Narrowed periodontal ligament; disoriented fibers.
2. Changes that may be produced by overfunction (within physiologic limits):
   a. Smaller than normal bone marrow spaces.
   b. Dense trabeculae.
   c. Wider periodontal ligament.
3. Changes that may be produced by overfunction on the pressure side (beyond physiologic limits):
   a. Compression of contents of the periodontal ligament.
   b. Hemorrhage and concomitant hematoma.
   c. Thrombosis.
   d. Compression necrosis.
   e. Ischemic necrosis and rupture of vessel walls.
   f. Hyalinization.
   g. Undermining resorption of the alveolar process, starting from adjacent marrow spaces.
   h. Resorption of cementum.
   i. Root resorption.
4. Changes that may be produced by overfunction on the tension side (beyond physiologic limits):
   a. Widened periodontal ligament.
   b. Hemorrhage and concomitant hematoma.
   c. Thrombosis and hyalinization.
   d. Apposition of alveolar process.
   e. Hypercementosis.
   f. Cemental and periodontal ligament tears (both may occur if occlusal force is of sufficient magnitude).

Prognosis. The accommodative capacity of the periodontium is the key to whether the resultant changes from occlusal trauma will be damaging. Certain factors may alter this accommodative capacity:

1. Age of patient. The accommodative capacity is at its highest in the young patient.
2. Gingival inflammation. The inflammatory process may hasten loss of the alveolar process and enhance the effects of excessive occlusal force on the periodontium.
3. Systemic conditions. These alter tissue responses to occlusal stress with the result that delayed healing may occur and the capacity to withstand forces is lessened.
4. Amount of remaining alveolar process. Loss of supporting bone may cause normally physiologic occlusal forces to become traumatic. The less remaining bone, the less is the accommodative capacity of the periodontium.
5. Force
   a. Direction. Those forces not directed along the long axes of the teeth are most detrimental (torquing forces).
   b. Distribution. Forces are more destructive when concentrated on a few teeth than when distributed over many.
   c. Duration. Forces that are continuous, as in clenching and grinding habits, are potentially more destructive.
   d. Frequency. The more frequent the force, the greater is the opportunity for damage.
   e. Intensity.

The clinician should always be mindful that, regardless of its direction, distribution, duration, frequency, or intensity, what really determines whether a force is traumatic is whether it produces destructive changes in the periodontium or within the stomatognathic system.

Radiographic Survey

Radiographs are indispensable aids in the diagnosis of periodontal disease, but they alone are not diagnostic. Radiographic interpretation should be considered along with clinical data to establish a final, accurate diagnosis. Each diagnostic regimen serves to monitor the accuracy of the other.

There are certain general requirements of a complete radiographic survey.

1. These film series should be included. Full-mouth periapical series and four-film periodontal bite-wing series. Panoramic radiographs are useful as an adjunct.
2. High quality radiographs. Films should be technically adequate in density, contrast, and angulation, and should include all pertinent anatomic detail.

Radiography will demonstrate the following information (Fig. 5–7 depicts many of the features).

1. Root length and morphology.
2. Clinical crown-root ratio.
3. Approximate amount of bone destruction.
4. Relationship of maxillary sinus to periodontal deformity.
5. Condition of interproximal bony crests; horizontal and vertical resorption. It should be noted that the height of normal interseptal bone is usually parallel and 1 to 2 mm apical to a line connecting the cementoenamel junctions (CEJ) of adjacent teeth. When these landmarks are not on the same horizontal plane, the resulting angular appearance of a normal alveolar crest may resemble a pathologic infrabony defect. The astute diagnostician must be aware of these CEJ relationships, as well as of the dense appearance of healthy crestal lamina dura, to avoid unnecessary periodontal osseous surgery.
6. Widening of periodontal ligament space on mesial and distal aspects of the root.
7. Advanced furcation involvement.
8. Periapical pathosis.

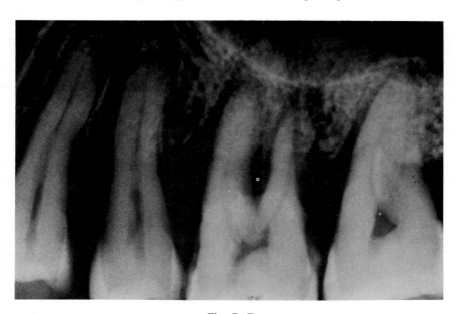

Fig. 5–7.

9. Calculus.
10. Overhanging restoration.
11. Root fractures.
12. Caries.
13. Root resorption.

Radiography will not demonstrate the following information (radiographs will not show disease, but the effects of the disease).

1. Presence or absence of pockets.
2. Exact morphology of bone deformities, especially tortuous defects, dehiscences, and fenestrations.
3. Tooth mobility.
4. Position and condition of alveolar process on facial and lingual surfaces.
5. Early furcation involvement.
6. Level of connective tissue attachment and the junctional epithelium (epithelial attachment).

Deposits Survey

A survey of the existing tooth-accumulated materials (TAM) is extremely important. To determine accurately the prevalence and distribution of plaque, it is necessary, even to the trained eye, to utilize disclosing solutions. For optimal usefulness in monitoring therapeutic progress, these accumulations should be measured and recorded repeatedly by utilizing a plaque index. The deposits survey is conducted last because the disclosing media used in this examination mask other important clinical signs, such as changes in gingival coloring. Some clinicians prefer to question patients regarding their current tooth-cleansing procedures at this time rather than during the dental history survey. The timing is unimportant, so long as the information that permits the clinician to correlate technique with effectiveness is obtained.

PROGNOSIS

Prognosis is a forecast of the probable response to treatment and the long-term outlook for maintaining a functional dentition. Hopeless cases generally present few problems in establishing an accurate prognosis. Neither do cases of simple gingivitis, which can be expected to respond favorably when local and systemic factors can be controlled. In borderline cases, however, the forecasting process becomes challenging.

Problems are compounded when the prognosis concerns strategic, severely involved individual teeth on which a large and complex restorative treatment plan often depends. This situation places a heavy burden of responsibility on the diagnostician under any circumstance. No formula can be established for such situations. Rules of proportional bone loss (such as one-third or one-half of the supporting bone) have been expressed in the literature as condemning a tooth for extraction. In practice, such rules are of little value. If adhered to rigidly, such rules may lead to the sacrifice of teeth that might have been retained in health. The difficulty with any formula or rule is that there are many exceptions. The best way of meeting the problem is to establish certain basic principles, criteria of judgment, and probable behavior patterns of doubtful teeth under the conditions in which they must function.

There are two aspects of prognosis: the overall prognosis and the prognosis of individual teeth.

Overall Prognosis

Overall prognosis is concerned with the dentition as a whole and is the basic determinant of whether treatment should be undertaken. It includes consideration of the following factors.

1. *Attitude of patient.* The success of periodontal treatment depends primarily on effective daily plaque control. Without patient cooperation and deep personal commitment and involvement in personal therapy, the prognosis is poor. This fact holds

true no matter how skilled the managing practitioner.

2. *Age of patient.* Generally, the younger the patient, the poorer is the prognosis. Given two patients with periodontal involvement of the same degree, it is logical to assume that the younger has far less resistance, because equal damage occurred in a shorter period. It follows that in a patient with weak resistance, healing and repair may also be impaired.

3. *Number of remaining teeth.* If the number and the distribution of remaining teeth are inadequate to support a satisfactory prosthesis, the overall prognosis is poor. Periodontal injury from extensive fixed or removable prostheses constructed on an insufficient number of natural teeth may hasten bone loss. Inability to establish a satisfactory functional environment for remaining natural teeth diminishes the likelihood of maintaining periodontal health.

4. *Systemic background.* The patient's systemic background affects the overall prognosis in several ways. When extensive periodontal destruction cannot be attributed to local factors, it is reasonable to assume a contributing systemic influence. The detection of systemic factors is usually extremely difficult. For this reason, the prognosis in such patients is usually poor. However, if patients have known systemic disorders that could affect the periodontium (e.g., diabetes, nutritional deficiency, hyperthyroidism, and hyperparathyroidism), the prognosis improves on correction of the disorder.

If periodontal surgery is contraindicated because of the patient's health, the prognosis is uncertain. Incapacitating conditions that prevent adequate plaque control by the patient (such as Parkinson's disease) adversely affect the prognosis.

5. *Malocclusion.* Irregular alignment of the teeth, malformation of teeth and jaws, and disturbed occlusal relationships may be important factors in the etiology and the progression of periodontal disease. Correction by orthodontic or prosthodontic means is often essential if periodontal treatment is to succeed. The overall prognosis is poor when relevant occlusal deformities are not amenable to correction.

6. *Tooth morphology.* The prognosis is poor in patients whose teeth have short, tapered roots and relatively large crowns. The disproportionate crown-root ratio and the reduced root surface available for periodontal support render the periodontium more susceptible to injury by occlusal forces, and any loss of attachment apparatus has a more significant effect.

7. *Recall availability.* It is increasingly evident that overall long-term prognosis is dependent on the patient's availability and his motivation to seek frequent maintenance recall visits, preferably at 3-month intervals. Patients who are unable to participate in a regular recall system, for whatever reason, are poor risks for periodontal therapy.

Prognosis of Individual Teeth

The following factors should be considered.

1. *Mobility.* Tooth mobility is caused by one or more of the following factors: gingival and periodontal inflammation, parafunctional habits, occlusal prematurities, torquing forces, and loss of supporting bone. Mobility is usually correctable, unless it results solely from loss of the attachment apparatus; this is not likely to be corrected. The likelihood of restoring

tooth stability is inversely related, then, to the extent to which it is caused by loss of the attachment apparatus.

2. *Teeth adjacent to edentulous areas.* Abutment teeth are subjected to increased functional demands. More rigid standards are required in evaluating the prognosis of teeth in such locations.

3. *Location of remaining bone in relation to individual root surfaces.* When extensive bone loss has occurred on only one root surface, the center of rotation of that tooth is more coronal than if all root surfaces were extensively involved (Fig. 5–8). Thus, leverage on the periodontium is more favorably tolerated than would be expected given the extensive bone loss on the one root surface.

4. *Relation to adjacent teeth.* When a tooth has a questionable prognosis, the chances of successful treatment should be weighed against the effects on adjacent teeth if that tooth were extracted. Unsuccessful attempts at treatment frequently jeopardize adjacent teeth. Strategic extraction is often followed by partial restoration of bone, improving support of adjacent teeth (Fig. 5–9; with permission from Dr. Ronald L. Van Swol, Chairman, Department of Periodontics, School of Dentistry, Marquette University, Milwaukee, WI.) This result is enhanced if the adjacent teeth are scaled and root is planed at the time of extraction.

5. *Attachment level.* The location of the base of the pocket in relation to the CEJ affects the prognosis of an individual tooth more than the pocket

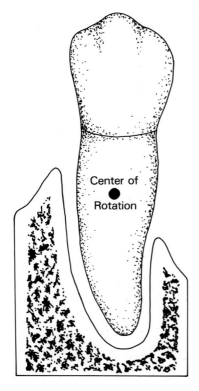
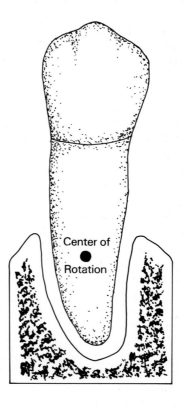

Fig. 5–8.

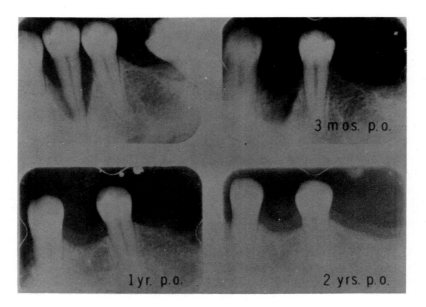

3 mos. p.o.

1 yr. p.o.

2 yrs. p.o.

Fig. 5–9.

depth. For example, a tooth with minimal pocket depth and extensive recession can present a poorer prognosis than a tooth with a deeper pocket and no recession and less bone loss. In addition, proximity of pockets to frenal attachments and to the mucogingival junction may jeopardize the prognosis unless corrective procedures are included in the treatment plan. When the periodontal pocket has extended to involve the apex, the prognosis is generally poor.

6. *Infrabony pockets.* The likelihood of eliminating infrabony pockets and their associated osseous defects is influenced by the number of remaining bony walls.

7. *Furcation involvement.* Bifurcation or trifurcation involvement does not always indicate a hopeless prognosis. Added support gives multirooted teeth an advantage over single-rooted teeth with comparable bone loss. Several factors influence the prognosis of teeth with attachment loss involving the furcation.

a. Extent of furcation involvement (see Chapter 18).

b. Access to the furca for surgical management. A narrow interradicular space offers a poor prognosis for new attachment procedures or root resection because of the close proximity of the adjacent roots. It also compromises the plaque control efforts of the patient. Generally, the more divergent the roots, the better is the prognosis; e.g., mandibular second molars have a poorer prognosis than first molar because their roots are shorter and the interradicular space is more constricted.

c. Access to the furca for plaque control. Generally, mandibular molars with furcation involvement have a better prognosis than maxillary molars with furcation involvement, because patients have better access to the furcas of the mandibular molars. Maxillary premolars with furcation involvement are poor candidates for therapy because of root morphology and poor access for plaque control before and after therapy.

8. *Caries, nonvital teeth, and root resorption.* In teeth mutilated by extensive caries, the feasibility of adequate restoration and endodontic therapy influences periodontal treatment. Extensive idiopathic root resorption jeopardizes tooth stability and adversely affects the response to periodontal treatment. In endodontically treated teeth, the periodontal prognosis is not significantly affected.

9. *Developmental defects.* Developmental defects, such as the palatogingival groove observed on incisor teeth and molars, present a poor prognosis for successful management. Root concavities observed in some teeth, particularly the maxillary first premolar, complicate the prognosis for surgical success as well as for maintenance after surgery.

TREATMENT PLANNING

After the diagnosis and prognosis have been established, treatment is planned. The treatment plan is the road map for case management. It includes all procedures required for the establishment and maintenance of oral health.

Periodontal treatment requires long-range planning. The value of periodontal treatment to the patient is measured in years of healthful service of the entire dentition, not by the number of teeth retained at the time of treatment. The treatment plan, therefore, is concerned with the entire dentition as well as with the individual teeth. Its principal purpose is to provide a healthy foundation for the future rather than simply to salvage those teeth that were affected in the past. It is directed toward establishing and maintaining the health of the periodontium

throughout the mouth, not solely toward spectacular efforts to "tighten" loose teeth.

The welfare of the overall dentition should not be jeopardized by heroic attempts to retain questionable teeth. The clinician is primarily interested in teeth that can be retained with maximal predictability. Such teeth provide the basis for a constructive total treatment plan.

A treatment plan should be developed to achieve the following objectives.

1. Reduction or removal of all etiologic factors.
2. Reduction of all pockets and establishment of minimal sulcus depth.
3. Restoration of physiologic gingival and osseous architecture.
4. Establishment of a functional occlusion by restorative procedures and occlusal adjustment.
5. Maintenance of periodontal health through adequate plaque control by the patient and regular visits to the dentist.

If the clinician can successfully attain these objectives, most cases of periodontal disease can be arrested on a long-term basis.

Order of Treatment

The detailed treatment plan must be based on the patient's dental and medical histories, emotional status, clinical and radiographic examinations, and the other factors that have been mentioned. Treatment plans, therefore, have many variations, but in general all consist of four phases: initial preparation, surgical therapy, restorative treatment, and maintenance.

Initial Preparation

This phase usually includes the following steps.

1. *Premedication.* Attention must be given to the need for premedication for subacute bacterial endocarditis, heart disease, hypertension, and

other systemic conditions, as well as preoperative sedation, when indicated.

2. *Emergency care.* Immediate treatment of periodontal abscesses, acute necrotizing ulcerative gingivitis, large carious lesions, etc.

3. *Patient instruction and motivation.* The patient learns personal plaque control procedures. Success depends primarily on the patient's willingness to participate as a serious co-therapist.

4. *Root detoxification (scaling and root planing).* Performed to remove calculus and contaminated cementum. This enables the patient to begin a program of personal plaque control as early as possible.

5. *Extraction of teeth.* Teeth with a hopeless prognosis and those whose removal will improve prognosis of adjacent teeth are extracted.

6. *Removal of overhanging restorations and other plaque-retentive areas.*

7. *Minor tooth movement.*

8. *Temporary stabilization.* This may be required to facilitate overall treatment or to aid in determining the prognosis of certain teeth.

9. *Preliminary occlusal adjustment and odontoplasty (if indicated).* Obvious gross occlusal abnormalities (plunger cusps, initial prematurities, defective marginal ridges) should be evaluated early in treatment and corrected, if necessary.

10. *Evaluation of results.* Elimination of etiologic factors may produce sufficient improvement to permit modification of the original treatment plan. In this sense, the initial preparation may actually be complete and satisfactory therapy. The patient's attitude toward plaque control responsibility is also evaluated. Additional instruction may be required, even though the patient is making a sincere effort to practice recommended techniques. On the other hand, a patient's failure to cooperate in this critical area should prompt the dentist to modify, limit, or terminate the course of treatment at this point.

Surgical Therapy

This phase of treatment includes procedures designed to reduce the pocket by resection, the relocation of the gingival margin, or the use of new attachment procedures. This phase may also include surgical procedures for the correction of mucogingival defects.

Restorative Treatment

The restorative phase usually involves definitive occlusal adjustment, operative dentistry, replacement of missing teeth by fixed and/or removable prostheses, and permanent splinting, when indicated.

Maintenance

Patients are carried in the maintenance phase for a lifetime. Most patients who have been treated for moderate to advanced periodontitis require maintenance at least every 3 months. The length of time between recall appointments is dictated by the level of disease control accomplished by patients during the interval between recall visits. This phase of therapy is often downgraded by both patient and practitioner yet it spells the difference between long-term success and failure.

CHAPTER 6

Plaque Control

As discussed in Chapter 1, periodontal disease is a bacterial infection. Many local factors influence its initiation, but inadequate plaque control overshadows all factors. In study after study, the worldwide prevalence and severity of inflammatory periodontal diseases are associated with bacteral plaque, calculus, oral debris, and poor oral hygiene. Neglect is the principal cause of bacterial plaque accumulation; neglect on the part of the patient to remove plaque, to seek dental treatment, to remove plaque after periodontal therapy, and to continue with their professional maintenance therapy, thereby permitting disease to continue.

Establishment of plaque control is an absolute requisite for the successful treatment and prevention of inflammatory periodontal disease. This requisite is true for all patients, but especially for those whose oral tissues have demonstrated low resistance to microorganisms. Such patients must be meticulous in their plaque control. Effective plaque control requires that the patient have comprehension and motivation, manual dexterity, and reasonable access to all tooth surfaces. Absence of even one of these requirements will compromise treatment.

Patients become involved in their treatment when they decide to accept all responsibility for daily control of plaque on a long-term basis. Their involvement is expressed by the action they take to remove developing bacterial plaque every day. The questiion is, "What action is to be taken?" Almost all of the various plaque control devices have their uses, depending on conditions present in the individual mouth. Generally speaking any action is desirable if it is effective, safe, and practical. Regardless of the devices and techniques prescribed, patients must strive to make their actions habitual.

EFFECTIVENESS

Effectiveness implies adequate cleaning of every surface of every tooth. Patients who brush frequently and manage to cleanse the occlusal and facial surfaces, from premolar to premolar, will benefit in those areas. Many other surfaces may remain uncleansed, however, and the contiguous soft tissues will continue to be exposed to the destructive agents of bacterial plaque.

Many of these patients think their brushing is effective, and express surprise when their own ineffectiveness is demonstrated. They may simply not be aware of all the surfaces that need cleaning. They may never have thought about, or may never have been told of, the need and methods for cleaning the proximal or lingual surfaces of their lower molars. They may actually be unaware of what they should accomplish. Their only exposure to instruction in plaque control may have consisted of a pat on the back and a friendly exhortation to "brush your teeth three times a day." For that matter, they probably have no understanding of the nature of plaque.

One requirement for effective action is that the patient understand what needs to be accomplished. Another requirement is that the accomplishment be realized. Unfortunately, there is no simple way to remove bacterial plaque other than to scrub or rub it off with bristles of a brush; with fibers of floss, tape, yarn, or gauze; or with a toothpick or interdental stimulator. As yet, no agent is available that will totally prevent plaque formation or totally remove bacterial colonies once they have formed.

The effectiveness of any method of plaque control also depends on whether the surfaces to be cleansed may be reached with the cleaning device. Tooth surfaces adjacent to shallow sulci are usually accessible to cleaning devices, whereas tooth surfaces adjacent to periodontal pockets are not. Obviously, there is less tooth surface to be cleansed in the healthy situation, and fewer concavities are exposed to plaque formation. In other words, as pockets deepen, additional concave root surfaces become available for bacterial colonization; cleansing difficulties increase. In recession or after surgery, more root surface is exposed. Although more root exposure complicates oral hygiene, the exposed root is at least accessible for oral hygiene measures.

These problematic surfaces continually challenge the patient's efforts to control plaque. The mesial concavity of the maxillary first premolar, for example, requires meticulous attention by the postsurgical patient. Furcations and developmental grooves of roots can also frustrate efforts of the most determined individual. When evaluating a patient's effectiveness in controlling plaque, one must consider these difficult areas and the possibility that the patient simply cannot adequately control infection in such areas. The patient should be made aware that although complete control of the disease in such areas may be impossible, reasonable effort, in conjunction with periodic professional maintenance, may significantly retard or stabilize the disease process. These considerations further emphasize the desirability of establishing plaque control before disease occurs. Generally, the effectiveness of plaque-control procedures is determined by application of the following criteria.

1. Minimal plaque formation, determined from a plaque index.
2. Absence of bleeding on probing.
3. Physiologic color and consistency of gingival tissue.

SAFETY

The effectiveness of the plaque-control procedure must be weighed against its safety. Any procedure that is inherently destructive should be avoided. Long back-and-forth strokes with a hard bristle brush, for example, can result in abrasive destruction of the gingiva and teeth. Toothpicks, improperly used, can destroy the papillae. Anytime a patient presents with damage resulting from plaque-control techniques, the patient must be counseled and the technique should be modified.

PRACTICALITY

A safe and effective method of removing plaque is of no value unless it is practical; this depends on the ability and the attitudes of the patient involved. A good rule for prescribing plaque-control techniques is the "KIS principle" (keep it simple). A complicated routine may be practical for a patient with good manual dexterity and zeal, but it is highly impractical for a truly uncoordinated person. If presented immediately in its entirety, the routine may seem impractical for a patient who has some skepticism as the result of past disappointments. If a complicated routine is necessary to enable this patient to control plaque, the practical approach would be to introduce the routine piecemeal. This gradual involvement during the initial stages of treatment may overcome the patient's skepticism as results become evident.

PLAQUE-CONTROL PROCEDURES

Brushing

For a thorough discussion of the many different methods of brushing, the reader is referred to current textbooks on periodontics. The sulcular (Bass) method is considered in this chapter as the preferred method for two reasons. 1) It is safe and relatively effective. 2) More and more practitioners who have had opportunities to make critical evaluations of all methods of brushing find that the best results are obtained with this method.

The sulcular tooth brushing technique was designed to remove bacterial plaque from facial and lingual sulcular spaces. If practiced effectively, the method results in the cleansing of the tooth-gingival interface—the critical area in periodontal disease. Cleansing is accomplished by directing the bristles of a soft brush into the sulcus and moving the brush back and forth in short, almost vibratory strokes (Fig. 6–1). The occlusal surfaces are cleaned by back-and-forth scrubbing.

Another important part of the sulcular method is the cleansing of the proximal surfaces with dental floss. Proximal cleansing must be accomplished if plaque is to be controlled. Unfortunately, little more than lip service has been given to proximal cleaning. Most patients who are aware of their disease and of its cause, and who are interested in arresting it, recognize the necessity for proximal cleans-

ing when the need is explained by a motivated dentist.

Manual Toothbrushes. Toothbrushes vary in size, shape, bristle hardness, arrangement, and length. There are a number of good brushes on the market and the astute clinician selects a brush that fits the patient rather than fitting all patients to the same brush. Generally, a brush with a straight handle and multitufted, medium soft, nylon bristles with rounded ends is preferable for sulcular cleaning. Smaller brushes are capable of reaching more areas than larger brushes. Patients should be advised that all toothbrushes should be replaced periodically before bristles become frayed and lose their shape.

Electric-Powered Toothbrushes. Electrically powered toothbrushes are available to the patient. However, a brush with only an arctuating stroke is not suited for sulcular cleansing; a reciprocating action brush is needed. A brush is available that offers both types of motion. It also comes with various attachments that are valuable aids in cleaning inaccessible areas.

The electrically powered brush is positioned exactly as a hand brush. A patient is instructed to permit the bristles to work subgingivally and interproximally, brushing only one or two teeth at each brush position. It is often difficult to position even the smallest brush head, manual or electric, effectively on the palatal and lingual surfaces. The electric brush can be used effectively in these areas by placing the heel of the brush (last row only) between the gingiva and the tooth and allowing the reciprocating action to clean the tooth and sulcus as shown in Figure 6–2.

Manual Versus Power Brushing. Numerous studies have been reported concerning the effectiveness of manual and powered brushes. Probably the most important conclusions to be reached are first, that a motivated, dexterous patient can produce effective results with either

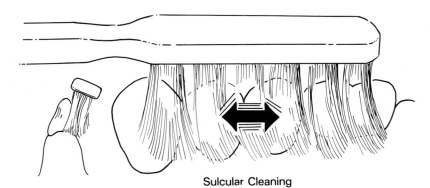

Sulcular Cleaning

Fig. 6–1.

kind; and second, that patients with limited dexterity can generally do better with a power brush. When patients demonstrate the ability to use a manual brush effectively or require only minor modifications in technique, there is no need to switch. When they have attempted a number of manual techniques over the years and have been unable to master one, consider the electric brush. It is often more rewarding, dentally and psychologically, to introduce an entirely new concept of

tooth cleansing, such as the electric brush, than to attempt to break bad habits that have occurred over the years with a manual brush.

Devices for Proximal Cleansing

Floss and Tape (waxed, unwaxed). Many patients, when they hear the term dental floss, immediately think of food caught between the teeth. Being uninformed, they have no conception of how to clean proximal surfaces and must be instructed

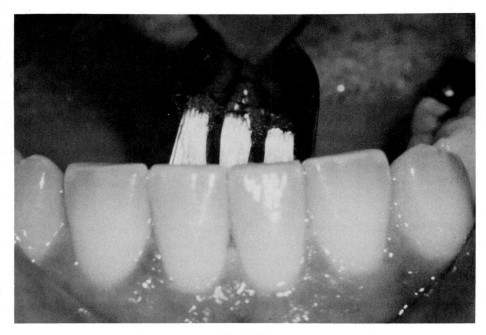

Fig. 6–2.

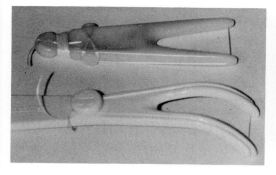

Fig. 6–3.

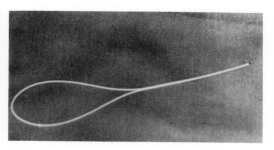

Fig. 6–4.

in what they are to accomplish, why, how, and with what devices. Dental floss and tape, either waxed or unwaxed, are equally effective for cleansing proximal surfaces.

The use of floss presents certain dangers that should be explained to the patient. Popping floss between contact areas of adjacent teeth can lacerate papilla. Damage can be avoided by keeping the hands close together, using only a short zone of floss, exercising control, and sliding the floss back and forth between the contact areas while pressing apically. The floss-holding devices shown in Figure 6–3 have proven effective for some patients who have difficulty in guiding floss with their fingers. Other individuals find it easier to tie the two ends together to form a circle, taking up the slack by wrapping the floss around a finger. This technique improves their ability to control the floss. Patients with fixed splinting of the teeth are faced with a difficult problem of access to the interproximal region. Floss can be threaded through embrasures by commercially available devices, such as the one shown in Figure 6–4. Removing floss in a straight occlusal direction can severely test the retention of restorations when contacts are tight. This problem can be alleviated if the patient pulls one free end of the floss through the interproximal space or pulls the floss through the contact laterally rather than occlusally.

In use, the floss is pressed closely against the tooth and is wrapped slightly around the tooth (Fig. 6–5). The floss is then moved up and down against the tooth surface, rather than in "shoeshine" fashion, cutting plaque from flat or convex surfaces. Problems arise when proximal surfaces are concave and inaccessible to the cleansing fibers (Fig. 6–6). Such surfaces require the use of other devices.

Yarn. Two-ply white nylon knitting yarn, used in the same manner as floss, is effective in cleansing smooth and convex tooth surfaces; the patient may need to tie dental floss to one end of the yarn to allow interdental passage. New products, such as Superfloss, may be substituted for yarn.

Gauze. Strips of gauze, in 1 in or ½ in width, are particularly effective in removing plaque from proximal surfaces adjacent to an edentulous space.

Rubber, Plastic, and Wooden Interdental Cleansers. Rubber or plastic-tipped interproximal devices can be used as aids to clean proximal surfaces. Some clinicians believe these devices can be used to promote and maintain healthy gingival contours interproximally, if used as demonstrated in Figure 6–7. These tools are also excellent for cleansing exposed furcations. Some individuals also attempt to clean within the gingival crevice by using a fine rubber tip and tracing each crevice. Rubber-tipped stimulators are available as attachments to the reciprocating action, electrically powered toothbrush.

Toothpicks and Stim-U-Dents. These

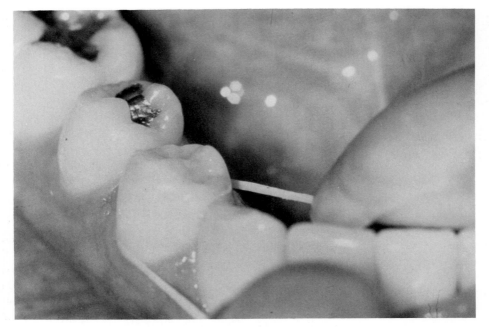

Fig. 6–5.

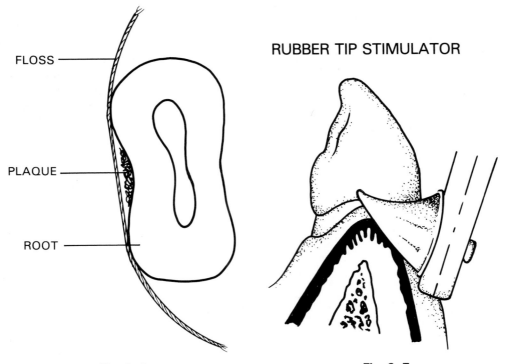

FLOSS

PLAQUE

ROOT

RUBBER TIP STIMULATOR

Fig. 6–6.

Fig. 6–7.

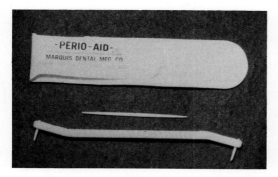

Fig. 6–8.

aids are used successfully by many patients who have been instructed in their proper use; improper use can result in damage to the papilla. Some patients have difficulty using these devices in posterior areas, but they are convenient to carry and their use readily becomes habitual.

Rounded toothpicks can be used effectively when placed in a special holding device (Fig. 6–8). The Perio-Aid is one such device. Each facial, lingual, and proximal surface can be polished plaque-free with the wooden toothpick. It does, however, require reasonable skill and effort. The effectiveness of all rigid interproximal devices is in their plaque-removing potential rather than through gingival stimulation.

Aid for Cleansing Inaccessible Areas

Single-Tufted (end-tufted) Toothbrush. This type of toothbrush is highly effective, well accepted by the patient, and safe in cleansing such areas as furcations (Fig. 6–9), concave surfaces, uneven gingival margins, malpositioned teeth, lingual and palatal surfaces, areas of erosion and abrasion, and those around fixed prostheses. Patients are instructed to trace the gingival margins with the bristles directed toward the gingiva and to hold the brush in each interproximal area, permitting the bristle to work interproximally and subgingivally. Inaccessible areas are dealt with individually. An end-

tufted brush can be used with the electrically powered toothbrush.

The Proxabrush (Fig. 6–10). This aid is useful for open embrasures where concavities cannot be adequately cleansed with floss, tape, yarn, or other devices. The Proxabrush includes a plastic or metal handle with brush heads of various sizes and shapes. The embrasures can be cleaned in a manner similar to cleaning a bottle with a bottlebrush.

Oral Irrigating Devices

Oral irrigators, whether of the pulsating or steady-stream type, are considered as adjuncts to the toothbrush for maintaining oral health. They do not remove attached plaque and consequently do not replace the toothbrush or interdental cleansing devices. Some reports indicate that irrigating devices may alter plaque. The relationship of this alteration to oral health has not been demonstrated. The water devices also remove loose debris from areas that cannot be cleansed with the toothbrush, such as around orthodontic bands, fixed bridges, and periodontal pockets. Recent studies have shown that irrigating devices are capable of reaching 3 to 6 mm subgingivally, displacing the unattached and motile microflora. The effect of oral irrigators on gingival health is still only speculative. Studies have shown that transient bacteremia may occur with the use of oral irrigators. The effect of such bacteremia in a healthy patient is unknown, but caution is urged in a patient at risk for bacterial endocarditis. The potential for transient bacteremia is associated with the use of all plaque-control devices.

Disclosing Agents

Disclosing agents stain attached plaque and make it visible to the dentist and to the patient. These agents are important for patient education as well as for effective plaque control. It is important that patients recognize the presence of plaque

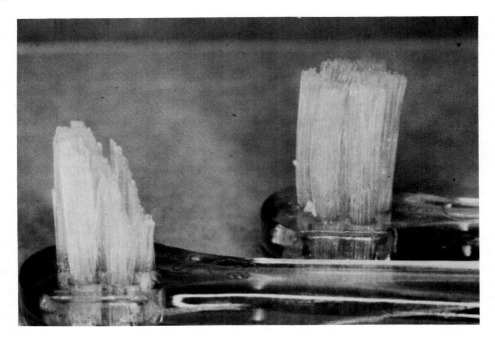

Fig. 6—9.

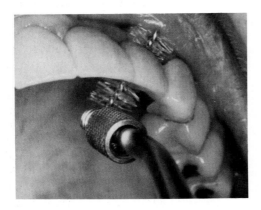

Fig. 6—10.

in their own mouth, and it is equally important that they know when the material has been completely removed. Numerous disclosing agents are available. Generally, solutions stain more intensely and last longer than tablets. Patient acceptance is also better.

Some of the agents available are: Erythrosin, Bismark brown, and FD and C No. 8 (a fluorescing solution). The latter requires the use of a special light or filter.

The Cleansing Routine

Plaque removal is accomplished in either a patterned or a nonpatterned manner.

Nonpatterned Method. In this routine, the patient is told, in effect, to "get the stain off." The patient is directed to rinse with a disclosing solution and then rinse with water. Then with good lighting and a mirror, the plaque-control devices are used to remove all of the stained material from the teeth and tongue. A mirror light and a mouth mirror are helpful adjuncts for viewing the stained plaque. When finished, the patient can restain to check the effectiveness of the cleaning method used, cleansing again if necessary. A disadvantage of this routine is the continued use of disclosing solutions.

Patterned Method. This routine stresses repetition of the same daily cleansing pattern with the hope that the action becomes habitual. For example, the patient is directed to use the proximal surface plaque-removing device first, starting at the last maxillary right molar and going around the arch to the last maxillary left molar. The patient then proceeds from the last mandibular left molar around to the last mandibular right molar. The patient next scrubs the occlusal surface with a brush, using ten back-and-forth strokes per quadrant in the same order: upper right, upper left, lower left, lower right. Subsequently, the patient uses the soft brush, applying ten short, vibratory strokes in each area, to cleanse all facial and lingual surfaces in the same sequence. When cleaning these areas, the patient attempts to reach a portion of the interproximal surfaces to ensure complete plaque removal from around the tooth. The patient is then advised to brush the tongue to reduce the colonies of microorganisms that may contribute to the reformation of plaque on the tooth surfaces.

Unfortunately, few patients are able to control plaque on their first attempt. They must be seen regularly, early in treatment, for evaluation of their efforts and for additional instruction, guidance, and encouragement. Patients' efforts at plaque control must be constantly evaluated from the standpoint of both effectiveness and safety, and they should be so informed.

TEACHING PLAQUE CONTROL

There are many approaches to teaching patients effective plaque control. No single technique has been devised that will satisfy the needs of every patient or that can be taught by every clinician. There are, however, certain fundamental principles that can be applied to virtually every patient.

1. *Keep instructions simple.* Remember, practicing plaque control is really an exercise in manual dexterity. The more complex the techniques, the more skill the patient needs to learn them.

2. *Do not teach too much at one time.* It is far better to introduce the new techniques a few at a time over a long period than to expect the patient to remember and practice a long list of procedures that, after a single episode, may appear complicated

3. *Encourage the patient.* Because of the varied abilities of patients, not every one will perform adequate plaque control at first. With further assistance and continued encouragement, most patients can be motivated to practice better oral hygiene. Do not, however, excuse lack of effort. One must differentiate between lack of willingness to improve and lack of knowledge and skill.

4. *Continue observation and supervision.* No matter how well the patient practices plaque control after the initial instructional program, the repeated professional evaluation is required to help maintain a high level of performance. The interval between these supervisory evaluations will vary from patient to patient.

5. *Be flexible.* Although you may teach a specific technique to all patients, remember that not all patients have the same problems. Crowded or widely spaced teeth, length of crown, presence of fixed prosthetic appliances, and physical disabilities are only some of the variables encountered. Be prepared to alter techniques, and be knowledgeable about products available for use as adjuncts in controlling plaque. Do not attempt to require patients to adopt your technique if their present methods are effective.

PLAQUE CONTROL BY CHEMOTHERAPY

Worldwide research into the control of plaque by drugs continues, with stress on antimicrobials and enzymes. The development of a harmless agent that would prevent plaque formation and remove formed plaque is an attractive concept that would have tremendous impact on plaque-related dental diseases. A number of drugs are presently under study, but considerable research is needed before these agents are available for general use.

In using a chemical to control the microorganisms of disease, five criteria must be met:

1. The chemical must kill or inhibit the micoorganisms in the laboratory.
2. The chemical must be able to reach the infected site.
3. The chemical must reach that site in sufficient concentrations to kill or inhibit microorganisms.
4. The chemical must remain at that site long enough to kill or inhibit microorganisms
5. The chemical must not exhibit harmful side-effects.

An oral hygiene technique, involving the use of baking soda and hydrogen peroxide, has been popularized by the non-scientific press. Although these chemicals may have antimicrobial action, numerous research studies have demonstrated that this oral hygiene technique is no more effective than oral hygiene with other commercially available dentifrices. Chemicals applied by way of a toothbrush and rubber tip simply do not get the chemicals to the subgingival site of disease activity.

Recent studies have demonstrated that a commercial "mouthwash" (which contains boric acid, methol, thymol eucalyptol, methyl salicylate and alcohol) is capable of significantly reducing plaque formation and gingivitis. This mouthwash is swished in the mouth for 30 to 60 seconds three times daily, after breakfast, and lunch and before retiring. The major complaints from patients are the taste and a burning sensation when a solution is held in the mouth. The value of a mouthwash is that it is commercially available and can be used by patients who cannot effectively cleanse their teeth manually. It is advocated *only* as an adjunct to regular control procedure, never as a replacement for tooth-cleansing procedures.

In considering chemotherapeutic management of plaque infections, it should be remembered that this option is for the future. Today, the only accepted preventive plaque-control method is physical removal of accumulated materials by tooth-cleaning devices. Therefore, successful control of the world's most common diseases, caries and periodontal disease, still depends upon effective action by the patient, who has been motivated, educated, and assisted by his dentist.

CHAPTER 7

Scaling and Root Preparation

PROCEDURES

Scaling and root preparation are essential ingredients of all phases of periodontal therapy. Mechanical tooth preparation usually includes scaling and root planing. It is often difficult to determine where scaling stops and root planing begins, and frequently, the two procedures cannot be dissociated.

Scaling. This is the initial procedure in which plaque and accumulated mineralized deposits are removed from the tooth surface.

Root Planning. This technique involves the removal of the root surface layer, which has been altered by disease.

Root Detoxification. This procedure is directed at rendering the root surface free of plaque, mineralized deposits, and plaque by-products within the root surface. This detoxification can be accomplished by mechanical, chemical, or a combination of these procedures. The use of chemical products to enhance the removal of toxic materials from the disease-altered root surface is under investigation. Examples of these chemical compounds include: citric acid, bile salts, and Cohn fraction IV. Future research may provide new and more effective products for root detoxification.

Rationale for Tooth Preparation

Supragingival Area. The goal is to obtain a tooth surface that does not encourage the accumulation of deposits and can be maintained by the patient. Scaling and polishing are the indicated procedures to achieve a clean, smooth tooth surface.

Subgingival Area. The objective of root preparation is to clean and detoxify the root surface to:
1) Minimize its contribution as an ongoing insult to the adjacent periodontal tissue.
2) Obtain a biologically acceptable root surface for tissue adaptation and potential new attachment.

INSTRUMENTATION AND TECHNIQUES

The successful practice of periodontics is centered around the skillful use of sharp instruments during scaling and root planing. These instruments generally include scalers, curets, files, and ultrasonic scaling devices. Calculus deposits can be removed by any of these instruments. Curets, however, are the instruments of choice for root planing.

Anesthesia

For most patients, *supragingival* scaling can be accomplished without anesthesia. Local anesthesia is indicated for proper scaling and root planing of *subgingival* root surfaces. It is recommended that practitioners use block or infiltration anesthesia and limit the appointment to a segment, quadrant, or one-half mouth. The practitioner can then accomplish adequate root preparation with minimal discomfort to the patient.

Technique for Hand Instrumentation

Basic Principles. Proficiency in instrumentation is obtained by adhering to general guidelines:

1. Work comfortably. Make the patient comfortable, but mainly, make yourself comfortable.
2. Follow an orderly sequence of instrumentation. This avoids omitting a particular tooth surface.
3. Operate with maximal visibility. When possible, it is best to have direct vision of the operated areas. Also, have a good light source. Fiberoptics are helpful in obtaining direct visibility. They can also be used for transillumination and may show small deposits that might otherwise be overlooked.
4. Obtain maximal accessibility. Use mirror and hands.
5. Maintain complete control of instruments. Stability is essential for effective controlled action of the instrument.
6. Maintain a clear field. Gauze and cotton rolls, frequent flushing with water, and compressed air may be used. Flushing is helpful in ensuring that no calculus or tooth shavings remain in the gingival sulcus or pocket.
7. Be certain all instruments are sharp. A dull instrument will merely slide over the thinner pieces of calculus, giving the impression that all calculus has been removed. Instruments must be sharp to be effective. Sharpen them after each use. Frequently, instruments require sharpening *during* the root preparation procedure.
8. Be gentle and careful. Do not confuse roughness with thoroughness.
9. Know the function of each instrument. Using the instrument correctly makes the job quicker and easier.
10. Use as few instruments as possible. You become more efficient and proficient when using fewer instruments.
11. Know the relation of the instrument to the tooth and periodontal structures before activating it. Put the instrument into place slowly and deliberately. This prevents undue injury to the tissues.
12. Check for completeness. Use explorers and probes for this purpose.

Basic Strokes. There are two basic strokes for scaling and root planing:

1. Exploratory stroke. This is used to determine the topography of subgingival deposits. The blade of the instrument is passed along the root surface or calculus deposit, apically, to the depth of the pocket. If any apparent obstruction is encountered during exploration, the blade should be moved laterally from the root surface and, if possible, gently moved further apically (Fig. 7–1a). This movement aids in distinguishing between a ledge of calculus and the base of the pocket.
2. Working stroke. Once calculus or roughness is located, it is removed by engaging the root surface and calculus at an 85° angle (Fig. 7–1b) and then deliberately moving the instrument along the root surface. This stroke is followed by a smoothing action done with absolute control (Fig. 7–2).

Use sharp curets with short strokes in a smooth, rhythmic, and continuous manner to accomplish root planing. There should be "stepping" or overlapping of areas around the tooth to cover the entire surface (Fig. 7–3). Care must be taken to avoid scratching or gouging

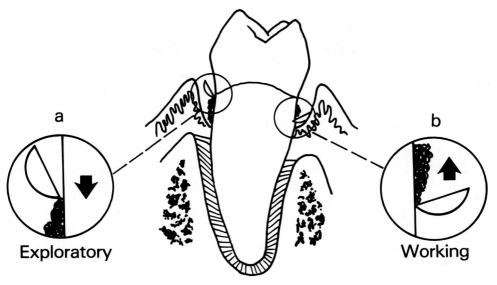

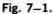

Fig. 7–1.

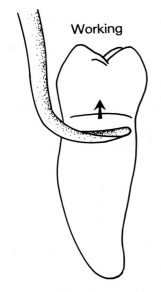

Fig. 7–2.

the root. The shaving action is continued until the root surface is completely smooth.

Ultrasonic Scaler

The ultrasonic scaler provides a fast and easy means of debridement with a high degree of patient comfort. The com-bined effects of cavitation by the water and vibration by the instrument against the tooth surface provides the force necessary to dislodge debris and accretions. No damage to soft or hard tissue will occur if light pressure and adequate water spray are used. Patients experience little or no discomfort as long as adequate water is used and the tip is kept in motion.

The inserts commonly used for ultrasonic scaling are the P-3, P-10, and EWPP (Fig. 7–4). The P-3 is excellent for supragingival calculus and can be used to remove subgingival calculus in the interproximal regions. The P-10 can be used anywhere in the mouth and is effective on subgingival calculus; it is used with any of the working strokes. The EWPP is best suited for debridement of deep pockets. It can reach areas that other instruments cannot traverse because of its similarity in design to the periodontal probe. The tip and corner of all inserts are potentially dangerous. Even a dull insert will gouge teeth and restorations if used improperly. Inserts should be inspected periodically to ensure that the corners and tips of the inserts are dull.

The ultrasonic instrument is highly rec-

ROOT PLANING STROKES

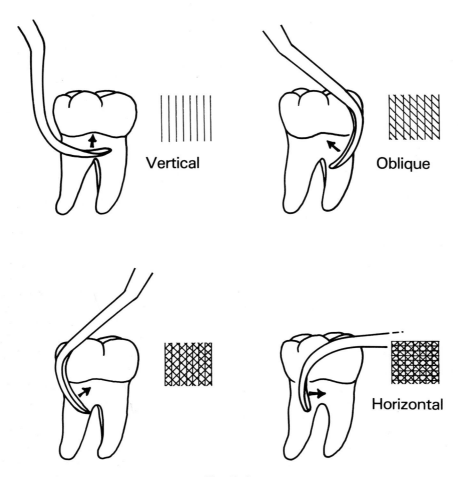

Vertical

Oblique

Horizontal

Fig. 7–3.

ommended for use in gross debridement, particularly in cases of necrotizing ulcerative gingivitis or acute gingivitis. The instrument dislodges debris rapidly, while the water spray clears the operative site. Some clinicians advocate the use of the ultrasonic instrument for debridement during periodontal surgery. A washed field with improved visualization is helpful during surgery; however, the water source from the dental unit often contains microorganisms that could be introduced into the surgical site. If the ultrasonic in-

strument is to be used during any surgical procedures, it should be used as a self-contained, sterilized unit with its own source of sterile, distilled water maintained in a sterile pressure tank. Even then, it is necessary routinely to check the tank and hoses leading to the insert for possible contamination.

The ultrasonic scaler removes deep calculus, but gaining access to the calculus is difficult, and there may be an absence of tactile sensitivity. The deeper the pocket, the greater is the chance of blockage of

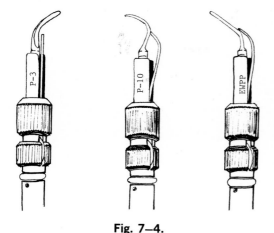

Fig. 7—4.

water spray to the tip, and, consequently, the greater the possibility of patient discomfort. Ultrasonic instrumentation removes the pocket lining, if subgingival curettage is the objective, and healing of the wound is as rapid as after hand instrumentation. It must be emphasized that the ultrasonic scaler is not intended for root planing.

Heavy surface stain can be removed with an ultrasonic instrument by using an "erasing" stroke and light pressure. A great deal of time should not be expended in removing stain that could be removed quickly and more effectively with a rubber cup and polishing agent.

It should be emphasized that the ultrasonic instrument is an excellent adjunct in periodontal therapy—but it is only an adjunct. One simply cannot perform deep scaling or root planing effectively with the bulky ultrasonic tip. It is highly recommended that a face mask and adequate eye protection be used by the dental team during the use of the ultrasonic instrument.

Polishing

Several commercially available, low abrasive, fluoride-containing agents are available for polishing the supragingival tooth surface with a rubber cup after instrumentation. Care must be taken that

products are selected that are minimally abrasive to avoid excessive loss of tooth surface.

A new instrument has been introduced that polishes teeth with the use of sodium bicarbonate propelled by high speed, high volume air to the tooth surfaces. The Prophy Jet has undergone extensive research as to its effectiveness and safety. Precautions are necessary when using this instrument on patients with sodium-restricted diets.

INSTRUMENT SHARPENING

G.V. Black stated that: "Nothing in the technical procedures of dental practice is more important than the care of the cutting edges of instruments. No man has ever yet become a good and efficient dentist until after he has learned to keep his cutting instruments sharp. The student who cannot, or will not, learn this should abandon the study of dentistry." Black, G.V.: Operative Dentistry, 9th Ed. Vol. 2. Milwaukee, Medico-Dental Publishing Co., 1955, p. 447.

Instruments are sharpened by grinding or polishing the surfaces that form the cutting edge of the blade until the edge is fine and smooth. Cutting edges may be formed by the junction of two plane surfaces, two curved surfaces, or a curved and a plane surface. Regardless of the type of edge involved, however, the basic principles of sharpening can be applied.

Sharpening Stones

The requisite for sharpening a cutting edge properly is to select the correct sharpening stone. These stones are made in various grits (textures) and in various shapes and designs to meet particular needs (Fig. 7–5). Sharpening stones may be grouped by design and method of use as either mounted or unmounted. There are three types of commonly used unmounted stones. The India stone is fairly

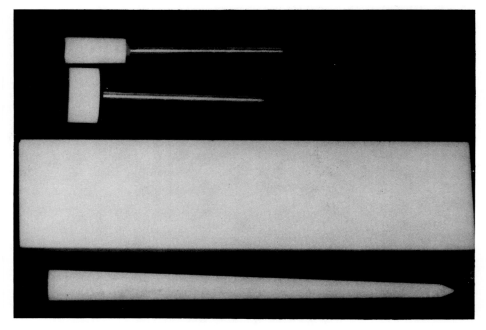

Fig. 7–5.

coarse; the Arkansas stone and the ceramic stone are finer.

Some mounted stones are inserted in a dental handpiece. The Ruby stone is coarse, cuts rapidly, and is used chiefly for preliminary sharpening when an instrument is dull. Mounted stones are also available in varying textures of ticonium. Other mounted stones are used with a specially constructed motor for the laboratory bench and with devices that maintain the desired angle. Honing machines are also available with specific sharpening attachment stones. Although the mounted stones are a faster method of sharpening, more rapid removal of metal can be expected.

Objectives of Sharpening
1. Remove the least amount of metal possible.
2. Retain the original angulation and shape of the instrument
3. Restore a sharp cutting edge.

Methods of Sharpening

There are many methods of sharpening periodontal instruments. Any method

is acceptable, as long as it meets the sharpening objectives. Two of the easiest and most common procedures are:

Method A. The instrument blade is properly positioned and is moved over the surface of a stationary, flat Arkansas stone (Fig. 7–6). A light grade of sharpening oil should be applied to the stone before the sharpening procedure.

Method B. The instrument remains stationary during this sharpening procedure. A lubricated Arkansas stone is positioned and is moved over the instrument blade to maintain the original design (Fig. 7–7).

Both methods of sharpening are followed by removal of the wire edge with a round stone applied to the face.

General Principles of Sharpening

The following method best describes the stationary instrument and the moving stone technique, but these general principles can be applied to all instrument sharpening. To ensure correct sharpen-

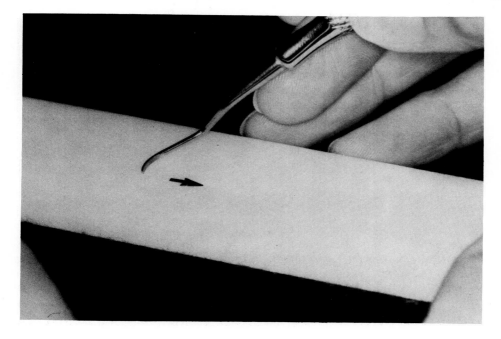

Fig. 7—6.

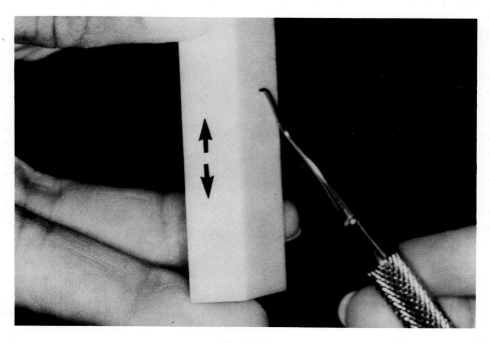

Fig. 7—7.

ing of periodontal instruments these guidelines should be observed:

1. Be familiar with the original scaler or curet design, including location and angle of the cutting edges of each instrument. This is helpful in restoring the edge without undue damage to the instrument.
2. Choose a flat stone that has been lubricated with sharpening oil (this preserves and protects the stone). Water is used as a lubricant on synthetic stones.
3. Stabilize the instrument against a table or cabinet top. Use a firm grip to hold the instrument and stone for complete control. The face of the instrument should be parallel to the floor (Fig. 7–8).
4. Establish a 100 to 110° angle between the face of the instrument and stone, thus producing an inner angle of 70 to 80° (Fig. 7–9).
5. Begin sharpening at the shank end of the lateral surface of the cutting edge and work toward the point of the scaler, using short up-and-down strokes of the stone. When sharpening a curet, sharpen around the toe to maintain its rounded form. Finish with a down stroke to minimize formation of a wire edge.
6. Wipe the instrument with an alcohol 2 × 2 sponge after sharpening has been achieved to remove the "sludge" of oil and metal shavings that form on the face of the blade.

Felt Wheel

A medium-hard felt wheel, 3 to 3½ in in diameter and ¾ in thick, is especially efficient for sharpening knives. Chrome rouge is applied to the wheel as needed.

Test for Sharpness

To determine whether an instrument has been properly sharpened, examine the cutting edge by reflecting light along the edge. A sharp edge is a line, rather than a surface, and will not reflect light. As the instrument is sharpened, the area of reflected light will disappear. The sharpness can also be determined by moving the cutting edge across your fingernail or plastic test stick until it "grabs". The fingernail method, however, is not always a true test for properly sharpened instruments.

All hand instruments require repeated sharpening. It is often necessary to re-

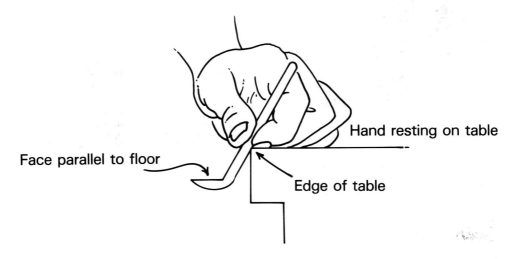

Face parallel to floor

Hand resting on table

Edge of table

Fig. 7–8.

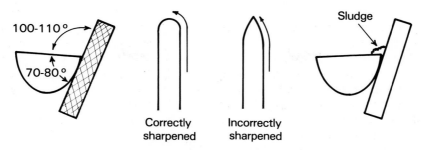

Correctly sharpened

Incorrectly sharpened

Fig. 7–9.

sharpen an instrument during treatment procedure. It is a good rule to sharpen instruments after each scaling and root planing before instrument sterilization.

Remember, if you scale and root plane with a dull instrument, you will waste time, work harder than you should, and have a poor end result.

CHAPTER 8

Tooth Movement in Periodontal Therapy

GENERAL CONSIDERATIONS

The importance of minor tooth movement in both prevention and treatment of periodontal disease is well established in the literature. The minor orthodontic procedure is often paramount in the preservation of a tooth (or perhaps of an entire dental arch), and a drastic compromise may have to be accepted if tooth movement is not considered. The objective of this chapter is to establish a philosophy of treatment, rather than a specific methodology. The subject of tooth movement in periodontal therapy is too broad for adequate coverage in the *Syllabus*. For additional information on this subject the reader is referred to standard textbooks on minor tooth movement.

Root Resorption

The possibility that root resorption may occur during tooth movement should not be viewed out of perspective. Many dentists consider orthodontic treatment and root resorption to be almost synonymous. When extensive root resorption does occur during movement, it is primarily a result of heavy orthodontic forces continued over a long time. The chance of extensive root resorption is slight when ap-

pliances are used with properly controlled forces.

Minor tooth movement requires only a few weeks or months. Cementum is more resistant to resorption than bone because of its relative avascularity. This fact makes it possible to move a tooth within the bone quite safely, provided gingival inflammation and other acute periodontal problems have been resolved.

Indications

Some of the principal reasons for tooth movement are to:
1. Correct tooth position to improve the function of the dentition.
2. Close an existing space where a tooth is missing, eliminating the need for a prosthetic replacement.
3. Enlarge a space or to improve the alignment of an abutment tooth for a prosthesis.
4. Upright or erupt a tooth to alter the soft and hard tissue topography.
5. Return to their original position those teeth that may have drifted or fanned out because of periodontal disease and/or oral habits.
6. Move a periodontally involved tooth within an infrabony defect, thereby narrowing the width of the defect

and improving the prognosis for treatment.

7. Improve esthetics.

Contraindications

Severe congenital malocclusions and jaw deformities, such as prognathia, retrognathia, and apertognathia, should not be treated by minor tooth movement. The same applies to discrepancies in interarch relationships and severe malocclusions that have developed during the growth period.

Considerations

Certain factors are necessary to ensure successful minor tooth movement.

1. The patient must be cooperative and must practice effective plaque control.
2. There must be sufficient room for movement.
3. The periodontal and periapical prognosis of the tooth must be favorable.
4. Periodontal inflammation must be controlled before and during active therapy.
5. The tooth must not be moved into a relationship unfavorable to basal bone. For example, facial or lingual movement off alveolar bone may result in dehiscences or fenestrations of the alveolar cortical plate.
6. Enough teeth must remain for sufficient anchorage and retention.
7. The patient must understand the reasons for the tooth movement, want the therapy, and be willing to cooperate through all phases. Unless the patient is highly motivated and is able to control plaque accumulation, minor tooth movement is contraindicated.

TECHNIQUES

Various techniques and different types of materials may be used to apply the

ELASTICS

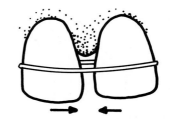

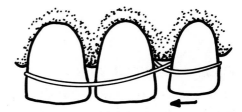

Fig. 8–1.

forces required for tooth movement. Some of the materials and methods currently used in minor tooth movement are discussed.

Elastics

Rubber elastics provide the simplest method of moving teeth in a mesiodistal direction. The elastics can be used singly in conjunction with a bonded adhesive system (Fig. 8–1) or with a modified Hawley appliance to move teeth in almost any direction (Fig. 8–2). The disposition of the elastics must be continually monitored and patients must be thoroughly instructed in their placement and daily management. Severe periodontal destruction can result when elastics are accidentally displaced beneath the gingival tissue. Elastics offer the advantage of the application of uniform force to all teeth that they span. They are excellent for returning anterior teeth to proper alignment when there has been drifting and spacing.

Prefabricated orthodontic force mod-

HAWLEY AND ELASTICS

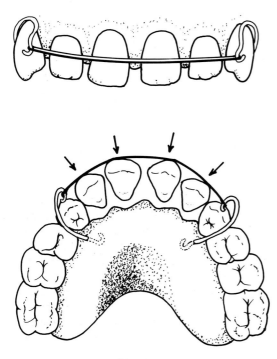

Fig. 8–2.

HAWLEY APPLIANCE

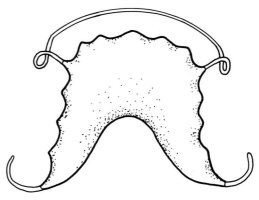

Fig. 8–3.

Bonded Adhesive Systems

Adhesive systems, which permit bonding of cleats, buttons, or brackets directly to the tooth surface, have added a new dimension to minor tooth movement. The bonded adhesives are particularly helpful for those clinicians who have never mastered banding techniques or who lack the equipment necessary to utilize metal bands. The various retainers are easily applied and have a surprising retentive capacity. The adhesive systems are versatile and are designed to accommodate techniques that incorporate arch wires, elastics, modules, or combinations thereof. The bonding material is readily removed with minimal loss of tooth structure. It also serves as an excellent material for splinting and retention, after orthodontic movement.

Hawley Appliance

The Hawley is one of the oldest appliances used in dentistry. Originally designed as a retainer, it has since been modified for tooth movement (Fig. 8–3). The modified Hawley appliance and the high labial wire are particularly useful for moving teeth in a palatal or a lingual direction.

The first step in designing a Hawley

ules afford the same advantage as rubber elastics but offer the additional advantage of a wide variety of sizes and shapes, which permits a somewhat more predictable application of force. Brackets are bonded to the teeth, and tooth movement can be accomplished by using essentially straight arch wires to guide the teeth and modules to supply the force. Buttons can also be bonded to the teeth and the modules are then attached to the buttons. The modules retain much of their initial elasticity, even after several weeks in the oral environment. This prolonged elasticity is a decided advantage over rubber elastics, which must be replaced at least twice a day.

MODIFIED HAWLEY WITH PALATAL CLEAT

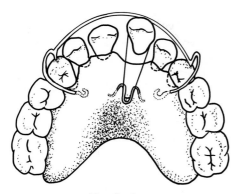

Fig. 8–4.

appliance is to determine the desired movement, and to incorporate the various kick springs, cleats, bite planes, elastic hooks, and other features in the design (Fig. 8–4). The acrylic resin should be carried 1 to 2 mm onto the lingual surface of the supporting teeth for stabilization. A horseshoe palate design is preferable to full palatal coverage. Retention of the appliance is derived from at least two clasps, placed preferably on the first molars.

The anterior labial arch wire of the Hawley appliance is usually 0.030 chrome alloy wire or 0.036 gold wire. A high labial arch wire may be obtained commercially. Usually, 0.022 chrome alloy is used for labial and lingual kick springs. The patient is instructed to wear the appliance day and night, except during meals and during plaque control procedures. Adjustments are usually made at 1-week intervals.

FORCES

The less force used in moving teeth, the less chance there is that the procedure may cause damage. Too much force results in overcompression of the periodontal ligament, with resultant necrosis and delayed movement. Generally, light pressure should be used over a long period

when a tooth is to be moved a considerable distance. Heavy pressure may be used for a short period when a tooth is to be moved a very small distance. Light force is produced by rubber elastics, medium force by the elasticity of metal (Hawley appliances), and heavy force by twisted wire ligatures. Whenever possible, the force placed on a tooth should be measured. A Dontrix stress gauge can be used for this purpose. The range of force is as follows.

Light force—2 to 4 oz (60 to 120 g)
Medium force—4 to 6 oz (120 to 180 g)
Heavy force—over 6 oz (180 g or more)

It is often difficult to gauge accurately the pressure exerted by some appliances. In any case, the patient is a good indicator of the degree of force that can be tolerated. The patient should be alerted that some soreness will occur for 24 to 72 hours, but that severe or persistent pain after this time is a danger signal. Instruction should be given to return immediately if the pain is intense, or to remove the appliance until an adjustment can be made.

Once the teeth are repositioned, the problem is one of retention. This period is when the periodontium reorganizes. Ideally, retention should be required only during the time needed for the periodontal fibers to reorganize to a new position on the tooth, and for the bone to mature. Retention can be accomplished by means of a bite-guard appliance, bonded acrylic resins, wire and acrylic resin splints, or a Hawley retainer. Long-term use of Hawley retainers is generally contraindicated. These appliances are potentially destructive to the periodontium and, if used for long-term retention, may contribute to periodontal traumatism, recession, and generalized breakdown. If it is impossible to eliminate all etiologic factors, or if tooth mobility is pronounced, a permanent type of splint should be considered. Teeth that have been moved from a cross-bite to a normal occlusal relationship rarely need retention.

The occlusion should be carefully checked and adjusted after tooth movement, and should be rechecked from time to time during the retention period. Most teeth that have undergone minor movement should be retained for 2 to 6 months. Teeth that have been rotated may require a longer period, unless periodontal surgery is performed immediately after they have been rotated. Severing of the gingival fiber apparatus appears to reduce the potential for relapse and the period required for retention.

RESULTS

The rewards of minor tooth movement in periodontal therapy are numerous. One has only to see the dramatic positive change in patient attitude, personality, and appearance to realize the importance of this treatment. Of equal significance, however, is the great potential for both prevention and management of periodontal disease. The severely malpositioned tooth of a young patient of today is a potential periodontal problem of tomorrow.

CHAPTER 9

Temporary Splinting of Periodontally Involved Teeth

TYPES OF SPLINTS

A splint is an appliance used to stabilize or to immobilize loose teeth. The following is a classification based on the duration and the purpose of the splint.

I. *Temporary splint.* This is used on a short-term basis and is usually advocated to stabilize loose teeth while undergoing periodontal therapy. A more permanent means to stabilize teeth may be indicated after therapy.

II. *Provisional splint.* This type is used for several months to several years and is used for diagnostic purposes. It permits the clinician to see how teeth respond to treatment.

III. *Permanent splint.* This is worn indefinitely to immobilize teeth and may be either fixed or removable.

Some of the temporary splints used in dentistry today and the reasons for their use are discussed in this chapter. It is important to present some rationale for temporary splinting and a few of the available techniques. Before the therapist decides to fabricate a splint of any type, the advantages must be weighed against the major disadvantage of compromising plaque control. Furthermore, the normal embrasure space between splinted teeth is often obliterated by the splint. Gener-

ally, when teeth are splinted, the patient must work harder and longer to accomplish the same level of cleanliness. Techniques should be employed that do not seriously jeopardize the cleansing of the interproximal space.

PRINCIPLES FOR SPLINTING

There are many types of temporary splints. The therapist should select one that will:

1. Distribute occlusal forces over as many teeth as possible.
2. Prevent the migration of teeth.
3. Not irritate the cheeks, lips, tongue, or gingival tissue.
4. Permit the patient to perform effective plaque control.
5. Remove a minimum of tooth structure.
6. Be esthetically acceptable to the patient.
7. Be prepared easily and economically.

INDICATIONS FOR TEMPORARY SPLINTING

Before temporary splints are discussed, it is important that some of the reasons for splinting be explained. Stabilization of periodontally weakened teeth is indicated so to:

1. Assist in the healing of mobile teeth after periodontal treatment procedures. Excessive tooth mobility may interfere with function and compromise healing.
2. Determine whether teeth with a borderline prognosis should be retained. If stability and/or adequate functions is not achieved 2 or 3 months after periodontal therapy, no further improvement can be expected, and either permanent splinting or extraction is indicated.
3. Reduce patient discomfort.
4. Stabilize teeth with a periodontal or periapical abscess.
5. Stabilize teeth that have been loosened by trauma.
6. Retain teeth in position after orthodontic movement.

TECHNIQUES

The following techniques are considered compatible with the practice of periodontics, and generally fulfill the principles for a temporary splint.

Anterior Teeth

Direct Bonding System

This method is effective in stabilizing mobile teeth, is easy to apply, is nonirritating to oral tissues, is esthetic, and requires minimal removal of tooth structure. Most importantly, it allows patients to accomplish plaque control more readily. Experience has shown that the direct bonded splint may remain intact at least 1 year. Some words of caution: direct bonding material may fuse with acrylic resin restorations, the material does not bond well to ceramics or gold, and complete removal of some of the adhesives (microfill resins) cannot be accomplished without damage to the tooth.

The teeth to be splinted must be isolated from the oral environment with the use of a rubber dam. The isolated teeth are then thoroughly cleansed of all debris and stains that would interfere with the bonding of the resin restoration. An acid-etching technique is applied to the interproximal areas of the teeth to be bonded, because this method increases the mechanical retention of the resin. A light-cured resin would be convenient to use because additional material may be applied and molded to the desired shape before curing. If unusual strength is not a requirement, however, an unfilled, autopolymerizing resin may be efficiently applied with a brush-bead technique. After the resin is set, the excess is removed and the restoration is finished and polished.

Unfilled resins have been shown to have adequate compressive strength, high resistance to fracture, and minimal marginal leakage. A drawback is its tendency to discolor, but this feature is minimal over the short time that this type of splint is usually in place.

Intracoronal Wire and Acrylic Resin Splint

These splints were originally designed to be used for short periods. Experience has shown that they may function for several years with proper repair. The technique for fabrication is as follows.

1. Prepare an undercut slot the width of a No. 330 bur and about 1.0 to 1.5 mm deep, midway between the cingulum and the incisal edge of the teeth (Fig. 9–1). Another technique is the incisal edge splint; a channel 1.5 to 2.0 mm deep is cut into the incisal edges with a No. 34 inverted cone carbide bur.
2. Apply a rubber dam and place wedges or other materials interproximately to limit the flow of resin. Place suitable liners for pulpal protection. Acid etching of the margins improves the retention.
3. Fill one half of the channel with

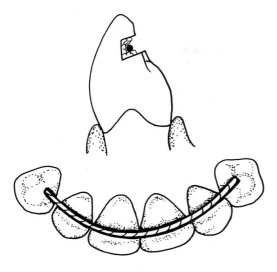

Fig. 9—1.

resin and lay a twisted double piece of 0.010-inch, dead-soft, stainless steel wire, or 40-lb test monofilament into the full length of the channel. Apply additional resin to the height of the preparation.

4. After hardening of the resin, remove the excess, adjust the occlusion, and polish.

Circumferential Wire Ligature

This method was a form of temporary stabilization used widely until the advent of the newer resin materials. Its use is limited to the anterior teeth and, unless carefully placed, it can seriously interfere with the patient's plaque control procedures as well as move teeth out of proper alignment. This method has largely been replaced by those for which direct bonding materials are used.

Posterior Teeth

Intracoronal Amalgam, Wire, and Acrylic Resin Splint

This technique is similar to the intracoronal technique described for anterior teeth. This splint has also been shown to function for long periods without breaking or contributing to the formation of dental caries. The presence of crowns or gold onlays or inlays may be a contraindication for this method of splinting and an alternative method may be required. The technique is as follows.

1. Prepare a simple undercut within the amalgams of the involved teeth mesiodistally with a No. 330 or 34 inverted cone bur. The preparation should be about 1.5 mm deep and 2 to 3 mm wide.
2. After applying a rubber dam, the gingival embrasures are blocked out with wedges or other suitable materials to prevent resin flow into the embrasure space.
3. A double strand of 0.010-inch, dead-soft, stainless steel wire is twisted into a braid and is fitted into the length of the groove.
4. Apply a microfilled resin until about one half the thickness of the groove is filled.
5. Place the wire in the grooves and fill the channel completely with resin.
6. Allow the restoration to harden. Remove the excess with appropriate instruments, adjust the occlusion, and polish.

Sometimes it may be necessary to remove all existing occlusal and proximal restorations or to prepare channels in virgin tooth structure. After protection of all pulpal and axial dentinal walls with a suitable material, proceed with Step 2 and apply the acid-etching technique with a suitable microfill resin.

The use of this technique offers several advantages: 1) This procedure can be accomplished in one visit. The use of amalgam may necessitate more than one session due to the placement of new restorations. 2) The enamel acid-etching technique and the use of an intermediate bonding agent improve seal and retention of the restoration. 3) The microfilled resin is harder and vertical stops are maintained due to less wear.

Bite Guard

This is an excellent temporary splint for anterior and posterior teeth. The guard distributes occlusal forces over all remaining teeth in the arch, is reasonably esthetic, does not require removal of tooth structure, and can be worn 24 hours a day—the patient can eat with it in place. Some patients experience difficulty in speaking clearly at first but with practice (reading out loud) this problem can be quickly overcome.

CHAPTER 10

Wound Healing

All surgery implies a disruption of the existing relationship of various cells and tissues of the body. Healing is that portion of the inflammatory response that results in the restoration of disrupted body elements into a new physiologic and anatomic relationship. It generally includes all of the following: clotting, granulation, epithelialization, collagen formation, regeneration, and maturation. An understanding of the healing process will permit the operator to design and execute a rational surgical procedure to support overall therapeutic objectives and to ensure that the patient's healing period will be as brief and comfortable as possible.

Periodontal surgery can be broadly classified into two categories: procedures designed to correct soft tissue defects, and those that deal with the management of hard tissue defects.

HEALING INVOLVING SOFT TISSUE WOUNDS

Excision of Gingiva (Gingivectomy)

After the removal of an excised portion of gingiva (Fig. 10–1a), clotting occurs with the formation of a fibrin clot overlying the connective tissue (Fig. 10–1b). Within hours, the connective tissue begins to produce granulation tissue (proliferating connective tissue characterized by mitotic activity in the fibroblasts, endothelial cells, and undifferentiated mesenchymal cells), which is soon covered by a great number of neutrophils, both on and within its surface. By this time, there is a base of moderately inflamed connective tissue covered with granulation tissue, a layered zone of neutrophils, and a clot—in that order. In the early stages of healing, epithelium begins to proliferate from the margins of the wound. Cell by cell, this epithelium migrates (at about 0.5 mm per day) under the clot and through the neutrophil zone over the granulation tissue (Fig. 10–1c). Epithelium continues to proliferate until it reaches the surface of the tooth, at which time the epithelial layer is only a few cell-layers thick. While this is occurring, fibroblasts of the granulation tissue produce collagen, which in the early stages of healing is not completely polymerized and is considered immature. By this time, the clot has been lost, having served its function as a kind of bandage. Proliferation and maturation continue until there is a multilayered covering of epithelium with rete peg formation. A gingival crevice is formed by coronal growth of connective tissue and by apical migration of the junctional epithelium (epithelial attachment). If healing has progressed relatively free from destructive bacterial agents, the lining of the sulcus is composed of a flattened, intact, stratified squamous epithelium.

Maturation of the collagen continues, with the disappearance of granulation tissue to the point that the formed collagen (the scar) is indistinguishable from the collagen fibers of the attached gingiva (Fig. 10–1d). Although clinically the tissue resembles normal gingiva within a few weeks, it will be a number of months before healing is complete and orientation of the fiber bundles occurs.

Even though the surgical procedure has not directly involved bone, there will be some osteoclastic activity on the cortical surface followed by osteoblastic activity. In other words, there is remodeling of bone to some extent, stimulated by surgcal trauma to the soft tissue. The remodeling is on a microscopic level and is not of clinical significance.

Simple Incision

When a sharp instrument cuts through gingiva, processes similar to those just described occur. There are superficial differences based upon the architecture of the wound.

If, after incision, the cut edges are closely approximated, there is only a small space between the wound surfaces to be filled with a clot (Fig. 10–2a). This clot serves no known function other than as a "plug" through which granulation tissue grows. Because the elements of the clot are ultimately resorbed, requiring cell effort and time, it is advantageous to have as small a clot as possible in this wound. Healing of this nature, by the union of granulating surfaces, is termed healing by primary intention. This is the rationale behind the continued emphasis on wound closure in new attachment procedures throughout the *Syllabus*. The better the wound edge approximation and the smaller the clot, the more rapidly epithelialization occurs, thereby sealing off the slower maturing connective tissues from the oral environment.

Epithelial cells from the wound edges proliferate between the forming granulation tissue and the clot, through the neutrophil zone, as previously described. When these cells join to form a bridge of epithelial cells through the clot (Fig. 10–2b), migration apically along the connective tissue ceases. After the epithelial

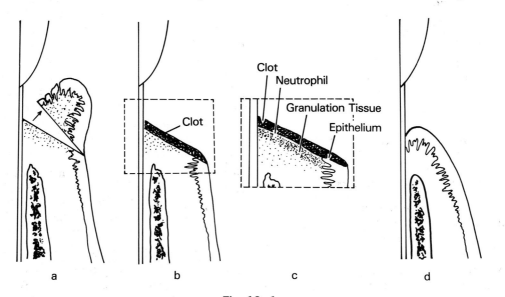

Fig. 10–1.

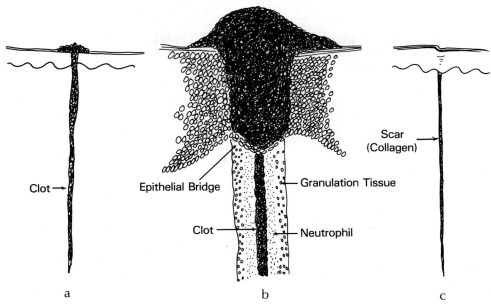

Fig. 10–2.

bridge becomes well established, the clot is sloughed from the epithelial area.

At the same time, clot dissolution is occurring within the depth of the incision, as macrophages remove the fibrin and as fibroblasts produce collagen. Once again, collagen maturation occurs with scar formation, which after a few months is clinically indistinguishable from the collagen of the gingiva (Fig. 10–2c).

It is also evident that in the relatively gaping wound, the epithelium will migrate farther into its depths along the cut surfaces; in fact, it may cover all exposed maturing granulation tissue and line the wound (Fig. 10–3a). In this situation, a relatively large mass of clot is sloughed (Fig. 10–3b); this is often termed healing by second intention.

Epithelial cells require energy for survival, proliferation, and migration. Their nutrients are derived by diffusion from the blood vessels. It seems that, in any given wound, the cells can travel only a certain distance from the capillaries, beyond which they lose their source of nutrition. The location of capillaries, then, apparently determines the route of epithelial proliferation.

Reattachment (Presurgical Level)

Reattachment can be defined as the reestablishment of a soft tissue attachment to the tooth after surgical detachment. If gingiva is elevated from a tooth surface, some collagen fibers will tear, leaving fibers embedded in and extending out of the cementum (Fig. 10–4a). If the tissue is replaced onto the tooth surface, a clot will be interposed between the fibers in the cementum and the wound surface of the gingiva (Fig. 10–4b). Some clinicians believe that if this clot is kept thin, granulation tissue will form, penetrate the clot, and permit the fibers extending from the cementum to unite with the new collagen formed by fibroblasts. In some areas, the collagen fibers in cementum will be lost; in these areas, new cementum will be laid upon old with the re-formation of Sharpey's fibers. Upon healing, the epithelial attachment may be at its original position on the tooth or it may have moved a few cells apically (Fig. 10–4c).

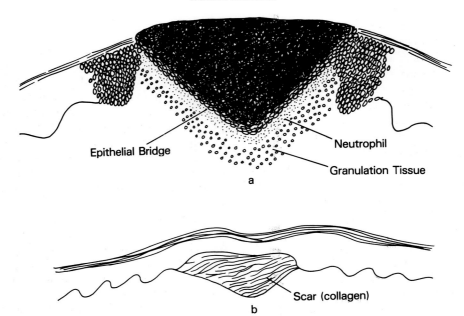

Fig. 10–3.

If a large clot is interposed (Fig. 10–4d), epithelium may migrate apically over the wound surface of the gingiva, resulting in an epithelial attachment that is considerably longer and more apically positioned (Fig. 10–4e). This occurrence is unlikely if normal care is exercised by applying gentle pressure for 2 to 3 minutes prior to placement of the periodontal dressing.

New Attachment

New attachment implies formation of new cementum, connective tissue fibers, and epithelial attachment on previously diseased root surfaces. To achieve a more coronal attachment of tissue to the tooth, cells capable of producing new cementum and collagen must have access to the tooth surface coronal to the present epithelial attachment. The epithelium lining the

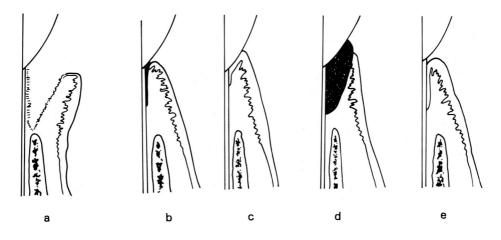

Fig. 10–4.

pocket prevents such access. This lining can be removed by excising the inner aspect of the soft tissue wall of the pocket. This procedure increases access to the diseased cementum of the root (Fig. 10–5b). If this cementum is removed by careful root planing and the wound surface is closely readapted to minimize clot size, cellular elements of the granulation tissue will resorb the clot and may produce new cementum and new Sharpey's fibers, and thus establish a new soft tissue attachment (Fig. 10–5c).

There is evidence that repair after gingival new attachment procedures usually results in a long epithelial attachment (Fig. 10–5d). Clinical experience and longitudinal studies suggest that this epithelial adherence is maintainable with little or no change with time. There is further evidence to suggest that by demineralizing the toxic cementum, a new connective tissue attachment is possible.

Confusion has existed for years as to whether new cementum will form on pulpless teeth or teeth with root canal fillings. Animal studies indicate that new attachment can occur on pulpless teeth, teeth left open for drainage, and those with root canal fillings, with the same predictability as for teeth with healthy pulps.

Open Wounds

At the completion of certain surgical procedures (gingivectomy, gingivoplasty), some areas of the wound will be denuded of epithelium and part of the mucosa. The type of tissue that will be produced during healing depends primarily on the type of tissue composing the wound and its borders. For example, a gingivectomy wound is bordered by gingival tissue and, predictably, gingival tissue will re-form.

After certain flap operations, areas of bone may be left with only a very thin covering of connective tissue. If gingiva originally covered the bone, then gingiva will re-form. If alveolar mucosa originally covered the bone, alveolar mucosa will usually re-form. Occasionally, and very unpredictably, an intermediate type of tissue may form, which clinically resembles gingiva (transitional gingiva). The formation of gingiva, however, can be predictably induced in an area of pre-existent alveolar mucosa if the apical and lateral borders of the wound are composed of mature gingiva. This gingiva seems, in some way, to stimulate the production of collagen fibers to the exclusion of elastic fibers. This result is the rationale for leaving gingival tissue on apically positioned flaps.

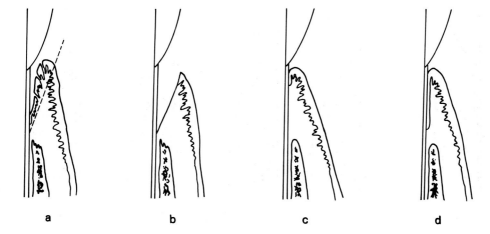

a   b   c   d

Fig. 10–5.

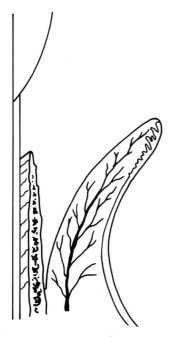

Fig. 10–6.

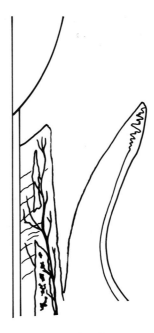

Fig. 10–7.

Flaps

A flap is defined as that portion of the gingiva, alveolar mucosa, and/or periosteum that is elevated or dissected from the alveolar process and retains a blood supply. Many surgical procedures involve the use of flaps of various designs. There are two methods of raising a flap.

1. Blunt elevation (full-thickness or mucoperiosteal flap) exposing the bone surface (Fig. 10–6).
2. Sharp dissection (partial-thickness or mucosal flap) leaving connective tissue of varying thickness covering the alveolar process (Fig. 10–7).

When flaps are replaced to cover the bone (whether in the original position or at a different site), healing is similar to that of a simple incision in that one connective tissue wound surface is placed against another with an intervening blood clot. The rationale and technique for the full-thickness and partial-thickness flap is discussed in Chapter 14.

Free Gingival Grafts (Free Soft Tissue Autograft)

In contrast to flaps, which retain much of the original blood supply, free grafts are completely freed from their blood supply and are placed at the recipient site. The vasculature at the recipient site provides all the nourishment for the graft. The problem with the survival of free grafts is one of providing nutrients to cells of the graft quickly enough to prevent their death in great numbers. For example, the outermost cells of a thick graft often die and are shed during healing.

The blood clot at the recipient site should be as thin as possible to permit ready diffusion of nutrients from the recipient site through the clot to the graft. Likewise, the inner surface of the graft should be as smooth as possible to reduce the "pooling" of blood and formation of thicker clots within the surface irregularities. Because the survival of the graft depends on revascularization, the graft must be immobilized at the recipient site.

Root Detoxification (Scaling and Root Planing)

It has been demonstrated that the removal of plaque and calculus from exposed root surfaces results in beneficial changes in the periodontium. This sequence of events is depicted in Figure 10–8. As a healthy periodontium (Fig. 10–8a) progresses to pocket formation (Fig. 10–8b), chronic inflammation of the gingiva results in depolymerization of some gingival fibers, apical migration of the epithelial attachment, and some loss of crestal bone. The gingiva itself is somewhat enlarged as a result of edema. Young vascular connective tissue is present within the gingiva, as are many lymphocytes, plasma cells, fibroblasts, and neutrophils (all the elements of defense and repair).

The granulomatous tissue has little chance to effect repair because of continued tissue damage from products produced by and from the microorganisms. If the local etiologic factors are removed by root detoxification procedures (scaling and root planing), and effective plaque control procedures are established, the disease process will begin to resolve. The edema will subside and the granulomatous tissue will be converted to granulation tissue and can proceed to repair with regeneration of gingival fibers. As maturation progresses, free from the effects of plaque, further shrinkage will occur until a condition similar to that shown in Figure 10–8c is reached.

HEALING INVOLVING BONE

General Principles

Bone undergoes remodeling throughout life. In health, osteoblastic activity balances osteoclastic activity. This balance can be disturbed by changes in functional demands on the bone and by disease. Furthermore, any surgical procedure affects bone to some extent. The severity of the change depends on several factors, including the type of bone (cortical or can-

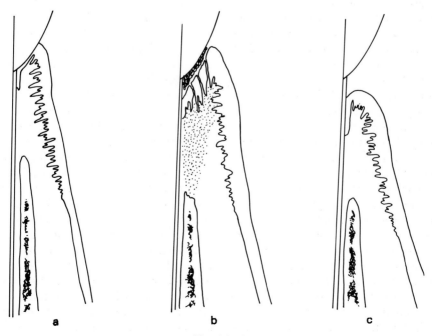

a   b   c

Fig. 10–8.

cellous), the thickness of bone, what is done to it during the procedure, and what type of covering it has after surgery. For example, if thin radicular bone overlying a maxillary canine were exposed during surgery and were left without soft tissue coverage after surgery, one could expect that during the healing process all exposed bone would be either resorbed or, more likely, sequestrated, and that little of it would regenerate. If interproximal bone, which is mostly cancellous, was treated similarly, some resorption would occur during healing, and the bone would then regenerate.

When performing periodontal surgery, one should remember that:

1. Bone should be covered by soft tissue after surgery, if at all possible.
2. The thicker the soft tissue covering over bone during and after the procedure, the less the bone is affected by surgery.
3. Thin bone can be permanently lost more easily than thick bone.

Thick bone, as seen interproximally, has sufficient intra-alveolar blood supply (cancellous bone) to withstand the loss of supply from the supraperiosteal vessels as a result of flap surgery. Conversely, thin radicular bone is almost totally dependent on the blood supply from these vessels (little or no cancellous bone) and can be readily lost if this blood supply is compromised. All canines, first premolars, and the mesial roots of maxillary first molars should be considered to have this thin bone. (These teeth may even have bony dehiscences or fenestration, as discussed in Chapter 1.) The thickness of the radicular bone over all facial root surfaces should be considered carefully in the design and execution of surgical procedures.

Infrabony Defects

Many procedures are performed to stimulate new bone formation for repair of an osseous defect. Figure 10–9a rep-

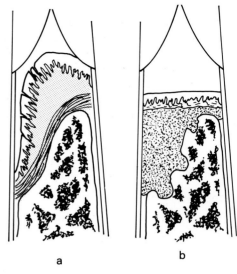

a   b

Fig. 10–9.

resents a mesiodistal section through the proximal surfaces of two teeth and the interproximal bone and gingiva. A chronic infrabony defect is diagrammed with the intent of illustrating three conditions common to most such chronic lesions.

1. Transseptal fibers are present as discrete bundles extending from the cementum of one tooth, sweeping obliquely over the crest of bone and its defect, and continuing to the cementum of the adjacent tooth.
2. A cortical surface may be present on the bony surface that forms the wall of the defect.
3. The epithelial attachment is apical to the crest of the bone at a certain distance from the base of the defect.

If a new attachment is to form and provide support to the tooth, it is necessary that cells produce new cementum, new collagen fibers, and new bone. To give reparative cells access to the area involved, it is necessary to remove the connective tissue portion of the pocket, the pocket epithelium, and the transseptal fibers. As this is done, granulomatous tissue within the defect is also removed.

After the soft tissue has been removed, if cortical bone is lining the defect, it should be perforated (intramarrow penetration) to permit quick egress of pluripotential cells for re-formation of the attachment apparatus (Fig. 10–9b).

Ideally, complete restoration of cementum, bone, and periodontal ligament will occur. Occasionally, however, only partial regeneration will result. The predictability of success for such new attachment procedures is discussed in Chapter 17.

Osseous Autografts

Autogenous bone grafts have been used successfully for many years in the management of osseous defects of the periodontium. The precise mechanism through which these grafts contribute to healing and regeneration, however, remains unclear. It has been postulated that the primary effect of autogenous grafts is osteogenic stimulation; however, these grafts are believed to act as actual bone producers as well as osteogenic stimulators, because of their high content of cells with osteogenic potential.

Another possible benefit of autogenous grafts is that they act as a mechanical block to the downgrowth of epithelium into the wound. They are thought also to act as a trellis (scaffold) for the proliferation and migration of cells and vessels within the wound. Generally, cancellous autogenous bone has produced better clinical results than cortical bone. This success may be due to the remaining vitality of cells within the marrow spaces as well as to the trellis effect.

Fate of Autografts

The fate of the calcified portions of autografts (and of other materials used) has been documented as follows.

1. The graft may retain vital osteoblasts and osteocytes and may be built upon by new bone. Such osteocyte viability is maintained only when the cell is close enough (within 1 mm) to a nutrient source, which suggests that osteocytes deep within a comparatively large fragment will die.
2. The graft may have no vital cells but may be built upon by new bone and later replaced by new bone.
3. The graft may remain as an inert, nonvital fragment, playing no apparent role in the healing process.
4. The graft may be completely resorbed during healing, having played no apparent role.
5. The graft may be nonvital, playing no apparent role, and may be exfoliated during healing. Exfoliation may occur months after the surgical procedure.

OTHER CONSIDERATIONS IN WOUND HEALING

Nutrition and Systemic Disorders

Healing occurs on a cellular-molecular level requiring the expenditure of energy and the utilization of nutrients as required for anabolic and catabolic activities. Any disorder that interferes with ingestion, digestion, absorption, or effective transport and utilization of foods will interfere with healing. Such disorders as diabetes, deficiencies in vitamins and foods (especially protein), and severe hormonal imbalances can be expected to retard healing.

Age

Age by itself seems to have no bearing on healing after periodontal surgery. General health seems to be of paramount importance.

Asepsis

Asepsis is a basic requirement for success in all surgery performed in the oral cavity. Periodontal surgery must be performed in a manner that will prevent introduction of foreign pathogens into the surgical field, which could result in infection and delayed healing. Sterile gloves, instruments, and drapes should be routine in the performance of all surgical procedures. Surgical mask and caps should be worn.

Healing Rate

It seems that there is a maximal speed at which various cells can clean up cellular debris, produce new materials, move through tissue, or perform reparative tasks. To date, there is no way to accelerate this process. Perhaps the best one can do is to avoid slowing the healing rate. To this end, such things as nutrition, trauma, smoking, alcohol, or other drug intake should be controlled during the healing period.

WOUND HEALING APPLIED TO PERIODONTAL SURGERY

A review of this chapter will serve as a reminder that there are many principles of wound healing that apply directly to the success or to the failure of periodontal surgery. A summary of the more important principles that have been discussed follows.

1. A gingival wound may appear normal within a few weeks; however, it will be a number of months before healing is complete and fiber bundles have formed.
2. The better the approximation of the wound edges and the smaller the clot, the more rapidly epithelialization occurs, thereby sealing off the slower maturing connective tissues from the oral environment.
3. In flap procedures, clot thickness should be kept at a minimum between tooth and wound surface to permit reattachment of connective tissue fibers at their original level or new attachment at a more coronal level.
4. For predictable maturation of gingival tissue in apically positioned flaps, gingival tissue should be maintained on a margin of the flap.
5. Thin free grafts placed on a recipient site over a thin blood clot afford an excellent opportunity for graft survival.
6. Plaque, calculus, and contaminated cementum must be removed for successful wound healing.
7. Bone should be covered by soft tissue when the surgical procedure is completed.
8. The thicker the soft tissue covering over bone during and after the procedure, the less the bone will be affected.
9. Thin bone can be permanently lost more easily than thick bone.
10. In the management of infrabony defects, it is necessary to remove all the connective tissue portion of the pocket (epithelium, transseptal fibers, granulomatous tissue). Also, the cortical bone lining the defect should be perforated to permit egress of pluripotential cells.

CHAPTER 11

Principles of Periodontal Surgery

The major goal of periodontal surgery is to create an oral environment that is conducive to maintaining the patient's dentition in health, comfort, and function for life.

REASONS FOR SURGERY

Provide Access

Surgery provides the clinician increased access to the root surface and alveolar bone. This access permits meticulous root preparation with the elimination of all hard deposits, contaminated cementum, and bacterial and tissue products from the root surfaces. Removal of toxic products from the root surface assists in controlling the inflammatory process. In addition, the reduction in probing depths after surgical therapy allows the patient better access to all surfaces of the teeth for more effective plaque removal.

Repair the Periodontium

In later chapters, surgical methods are described that are designed to restore soft tissue and bone destroyed by disease. This surgery consists primarily of hard- and soft-tissue grafting techniques to restore the periodontium to a state that approaches the pre-disease level.

Modify Bony Architecture

Osseous defects and deformities create aberrations in the physiologic contour of the periodontium that contribute to plaque retention and are not consistent with a state of good health. Contouring the bone to eliminate osseous defects reduces plaque-retentive areas and allows the patient better access to the tooth surfaces for more effective plaque control.

Reduce Periodontal Pockets

Periodontal pockets may not always be totally eliminated, but they may be reduced by a variety of resective and regenerative techniques (Chapters 12 to 19). The primary goal is to reduce pocket depth to a manageable level for the dental team and for the patient.

PRESURGICAL CONSIDERATIONS

Patient Consent

When the periodontal treatment plan is presented to the patient, the patient should be informed that surgery may be a part of that plan. The patient should clearly understand the benefits and the possible risks or complications of any proposed procedures. The alternatives to surgery should be carefully explained to enable the patient to give an informed consent to the operative plan. A written entry of the discussion and patient agreement should be made in the dental record.

Contraindications for Periodontal Surgery

There are a number of reasons for not performing periodontal surgery. The existence of certain medical problems could make periodontal surgery inadvisable. A complete and thorough medical history must be taken before the performance of *any* periodontal treatment (see Chapter 3). Excellent plaque control is mandatory for success of periodontal surgery. The patient must be informed, at any early stage of the treatment, that *no* surgery will be performed unless the plaque is adequately controlled before surgery and until the patient understands and is committed to long-term maintenance care.

The magnitude of the existing periodontal destruction must be considered. Surgery performed in an attempt to treat severe periodontal destruction could result in further mutilating the tissues, rather than restoring the periodontium to health, comfort, and function. There are many instances in which extraction of teeth is the treatment of choice in managing the severely involved patient.

There are some patients who prefer to forego surgery, even after the advantages of surgery have been explained carefully. The best course of action with these patients is to cease further discussion of surgery and to determine an alternative type of treatment to maintain the existing dentition.

No periodontal surgery should be attempted by a practitioner who does not feel capable of the surgical management of the patient's condition. The dentist loses no status or prestige in the eyes of the patient in referring the advanced case to a trained specialist.

Initial/Phase I Therapy

Initial or Phase I therapy should be completed before the final decision is made to perform surgery. Phase I therapy is one of the most valuable components of periodontal therapy. During this phase, it is possible to assess the patient's commitment to periodontal therapy, to observe the patient's healing potential, to reinforce plaque control instruction, to reduce the need for surgery, and to improve tissue tone which facilitates soft tissue management at the time of surgery.

Three to 6 weeks after completing Phase I therapy, the patient is re-examined thoroughly to determine what changes have occurred and what further periodontal therapy is required. On the basis of this examination, a decision must be made regarding which one of the three treatment options will be followed.

Option 1. The patient's plaque control is excellent and there is no evidence of active disease. In this situation, periodontal surgery would not be required and the patient would be placed in a periodontal maintenance recall program.

Option 2. The patient achieves an acceptable level of plaque control, but active disease that requires surgical correction is still present. Surgical therapy in this situation would be appropriate.

Option 3. The patient's plaque control is inadequate, even after many plaque-control instruction sessions. Active disease is present. Surgery should not be undertaken. This patient should be placed in a compromise maintenance program with frequent recalls. At each recall visit, a thorough periodontal clinical examination, plaque-control instruction, and scaling and root planing should be performed. If the patient's compliance improves, a reconsideration of surgery may be in order.

Anxiety Control

Most anxiety can be controlled by managing the patient in a kind and considerate manner. The periodontal surgeon should exude calm confidence in his/her ability to accomplish the surgical procedure. There are a few patients whose anxiety cannot be controlled without the utilization of some form of tranquilizing or sedative therapy. A variety of medications and methods are available for this purpose. Incumbent with utilization of sedation or drug therapy is the responsibility of the clinician to be thoroughly familiar with all aspects of the methods being considered.

Antibiotics

Premedication with appropriate antibiotics *must* be provided for the following systemic conditions:

1. Most congenital heart disease.
2. Rheumatic heart disease or other acquired valvular heart disease.
3. Idiopathic hypertrophic subaortic stenosis.
4. Mitral valve prolapse syndrome with mitral insufficiency.
5. Prosthetic heart valves.
6. Patients with joint prostheses.

The recommendations of the American Heart Association (Regimen A or B) should be followed for conditions 1 through 4. Regimen B is the treatment of choice for patients with prosthetic heart valves. There is no consensus on the best antibiotic coverage for patients with a joint prosthesis. One suggested course of treatement is 500 mg Keflex every 6 hours for 3 days, starting on the day of surgery. An alternative for those patients allergic to Keflex is Clindamycin (300 mg every 6 hours for 3 days, starting the day of surgery).

There is a minimal amount of evidence to support the concept of prophylactic administration of antibiotics to prevent infection after periodontal surgery. The use of broad-spectrum antibiotics to suppress plaque and to improve healing after bone grafting procedures has considerable merit. Tetracycline is selectively excreted in gingival fluid in a concentration two to ten times the concentration found in plasma. This high concentration in the target gingival sulcular area makes tetracycline particularly appropriate to prescribe after bone grafting. The usual dosage is 250 mg four times per day, starting on the day of surgery and for 7 days thereafter. Tetracycline should not be taken with food because of the likelihood of impaired absorption. In addition, this antibiotic may cause discoloration of developing teeth; therefore, caution should be observed in prescribing it for women in the third trimester of pregnancy, or for children with developing dentitions. Tetracycline is also contraindicated in patients with impaired liver and kidney function and those with known allergies to the medication.

Asepsis

It is imperative that periodontal surgery be performed under aseptic conditions. It is not possible to sterilize the oral cavity, but precautions should be taken to prevent cross-examination and to preclude the introduction of extraneous bacteria into the patient's mouth. All instruments must be sterilized and placed on a sterile operating tray. The operator should don surgical cap, mask, and gloves. A sterile towel should be clipped to the front of the surgeon's clinic coat. The patient should be draped with sterile towels and the patient's hair and eyes may be wrapped with sterile towels. Great care should be taken to ensure that nonsterile items are not introduced into the operating field.

Emergencies

The clinician must know and take measures to minimize adverse patient reactions to any administered medication. All office personnel must have ready access to the emergency cart and be competent in the proper use of emergency equipment. Periodic inspection of emergency equipment must be made to ensure that the equipment is in good working condition. Each member of the office staff should be currently certified in basic cardiopulmonary resuscitation. It is good policy to have periodic drills in emergency procedures so that each staff member will have the confidence to perform effectively in an emergency situation.

Anesthesia

Periodontal surgery is usually performed under local anesthesia. The periodontal surgeon should use the minimum of local anesthetic required to keep the patient comfortable during the surgical procedure. The clinician should be aware that the dosage, the method of injection, and the vascularity at the injected site have an effect on the patient.

The action and safe dose range of the anesthetic selected should be well known. The maximal safe dosage for lidocaine hydrochloride in a healthy person, when used with a vasoconstrictor, is 3.2 mg per pound of body weight. A 1.8-ml dental cartridge with 2% lidocaine hydrochloride contains 36 mg of lidocaine hydrochloride (20 mg per ml). By using this information, it is possible to calculate the maximal dose for a healthy patient. For example, 12 cartridges of 2% hydrochloride is the maximum that could be used for a 140-lb person (140 lb × 3.2 mg = 448 mg: $\dfrac{448 \text{ mg}}{36 \text{ mg cartridge}} = 12.4$ cartridges).

It is usually unnecessary for the epinephrine concentration to be greater than 1:100,000 (0.01 mg/ml) in local anesthetic agents used for periodontal surgery. The maximal dosage of epinephrine for a healthy adult patient is 0.2 mg epinephrine per dental appointment. Patients with severe cardiovascular problems should receive no more than 0.04 mg epinephrine per dental appointment (two 1.8-ml cartridges of anesthetic with 1:100,000 epinephrine concentration).

CAUTION: Injection of any local anesthetic in dentistry should be accomplished with aspirating syringes, and at a rate that approximates 1 ml/min.

SURGICAL CONSIDERATIONS

Surgical Plan

Before surgery, the clinician should carefully review the patient's radiographs and information regarding probing depths, amount of attached and keratinized tissue, and bony contours. These data are used to plan carefully the proper surgical procedure. Although a specific surgical plan is necessary, the clinician should be flexible enough to change the plan if an unsuspected problem is encountered during the surgery.

Instrumentation and Flap Design

Cutting and planing instruments must be sharp. Dull instruments traumatize tissue, complicate healing, and frustrate the operator. If dull instruments are found in a set, a sterile sharp instrument should be obtained before proceeding. Extra scalpel blades should be readily available.

Continuous awareness of the location of the cutting edge of a knife will prevent conversion of a flap into a free graft. Cells die when abused. This basic fact suggests a healthy respect for tissue during its manipulation. When a flap is being retracted after elevation, for example, there will be less trauma if the retractor is held gently but firmly against bone instead of against the undersurface of the flap.

Vertical relaxing incisions or access incisions extending toward the palatal vault or along the lingual alveolar plate in the mandible should be avoided. Incisions of this type, particularly in the palate, can interfere with the blood supply to tissue medial to the incision. In addition, the greater palatine artery may be severed if a vertical incision is placed in the posterior part of the palate. Hemorrhage from this vessel can be of major proportions. These incisions may be difficult to suture and often heal slowly with noticeable discomfort to the patient, especially those incisions in the mandible. These problems can usually be avoided by extending the initial flap incision to include a few teeth mesial or distal to the area of instrumentation. If vertical incisions are utilized on the facial side, they should be designed so as not to compromise the blood supply of the flap (Fig. 11–1). Also, vertical incisions should be made at line angles to preserve the interdental papillae for suturing and to prevent necrosis of the wound

edge; under no circumstances should vertical incisions be made over the midfacial (radicular) surface of roots (Fig. 11–2). If a periodontally weakened tooth is used as a fulcrum for elevation of a flap (especially a palatal flap), accidental removal of a tooth can result.

It is essential that good visibility of the surgical site be maintained at all times. Blood and saliva may be eliminated from the operative area with good aspiration or by applying intermittent pressure with moist gauze sponges and using periodic

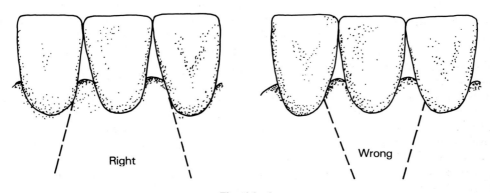

Fig. 11–1.

INCORRECT VERTICAL INCISIONS

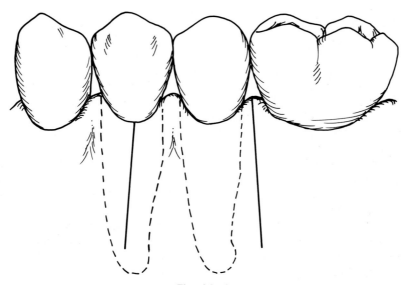

Fig. 11–2.

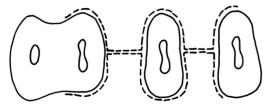

Fig. 11–3.

irrigation. The gauze sponges should not have a cotton fiber liner.

Bone contouring can be done with sharp chisels or rotating instruments. Caution should be exercised, especially if hand pressure is used, to prevent slipping of the instruments. If a handpiece and burs or stones are used, a sterile saline coolant should bathe the area. A fiber-optic handpiece is useful for improved visibility when contouring bone. Ultra-speed cutting should be done with the lightest pressure and intermittent contact.

Control of Bleeding

Bleeding may be controlled during resective procedures by putting pressure directly on the bleeding site with a saline-moistened gauze sponge. Bleeding control during flap surgery may be accomplished by replacing the flap and applying pressure to the flap with moistened gauze sponges. The pressure on the flap should be sufficient to overcome capillary or arteriolar pressure, but not be so heavy as to cause tissue damage. Many times, heavy bleeding occurs from the interproximal tissues after flap elevation. This bleeding usually stops as soon as all of the granulomatous tissue has been removed. Bleeding from a nutrient canal in the bone can be controlled by crushing the adjacent bone into (swaging) the canal with pressure applied by a metal instrument.

There are substances that are useful in areas where bleeding cannot be controlled by pressure. Thrombin-impregnated oxidized cellulose (Surgicel) strips may be placed over the bleeding site, with gentle pressure applied. These strips may be reapplied as necessary and will resorb over a short time. Microfibrillar collagen hemostat (MCH-Avitene) is another effective hemostatic agent. This material is a dry, sterile, shredded fluff, which is placed with a dry cotton forceps on the bleeding site as required. MCH is resorbable and causes no adverse tissue or systemic reaction.

The use of topically applied epinephrine is not recommended as a hemostatic agent. Epinephrine is readily introduced

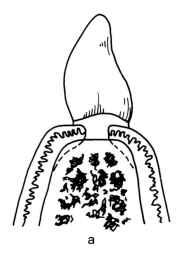

a

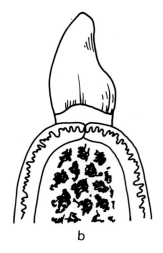

b

Fig. 11–4.

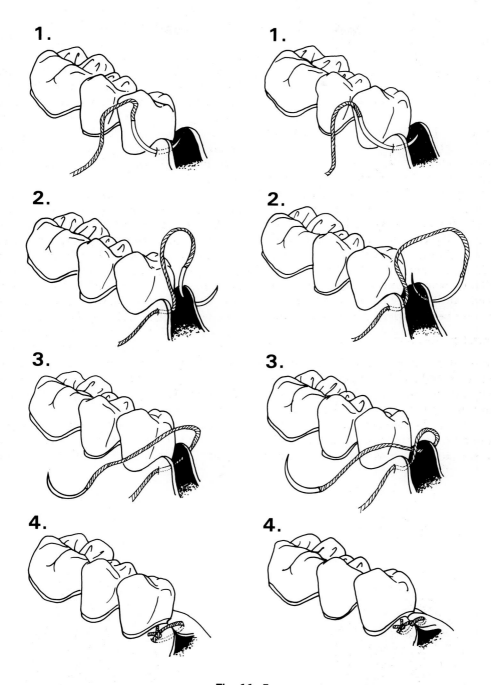

Fig. 11–5.

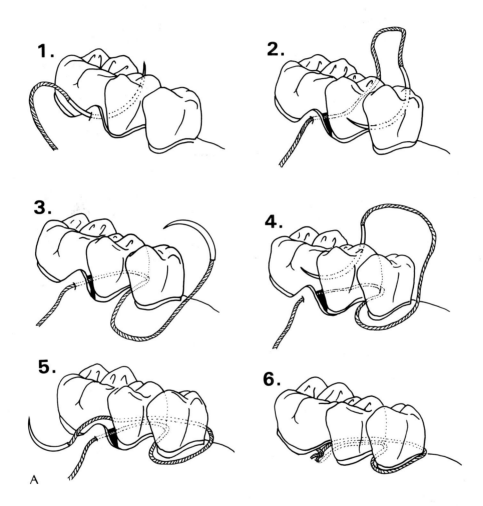

Fig. 11–6. A

A

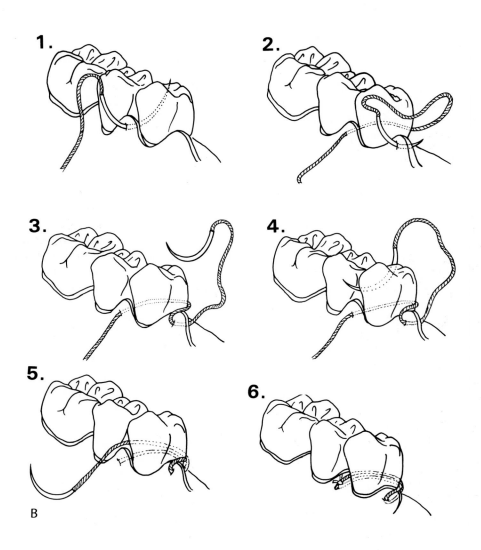

B

Fig. 11–6. B

into the systemic circulation and can cause significant elevation of blood pressure, cardiac arrhythmias, and possibly ventricular fibrillation. Patients with cardiovascular disease could be placed in an acute life-threatening situation from the use of topical epinephrine.

Bleeding should be stopped before the dressings are placed. The hemostatic effect of periodontal dressing is not great, nor are they adequate pressure dressings. Remember to strive for minimal blood clots in new attachment procedures. This goal is accomplished by applying gentle pressure to the flap or graft, with gauze soaked in saline solution, for 2 to 3 minutes before the placement of the dressing. When the patient leaves the operative suite, there should be no bleeding from the surgical site.

Wound Closure

Wound closure is important to the success of new attachment procedures and bone grafting. The flap should be designed to permit maximal opportunity for primary closure in the interproximal region. As much interdental papilla as possible must be maintained, which is achieved by utilizing a scalloped incision (Fig. 11–3). Proximal osteoplasty may be performed to improve approximation of the wound edges when performing new attachment procedures (Fig. 11–4)*a* and *b*).

Suturing

Suturing is performed to provide proper wound closure, to position tissues, to control bleeding, and to help reduce postoperative pain. As stated above, primary wound closure is necessary for successful new attachment and bone-grafting techniques. Precise suturing is imperative in mucogingival surgical procedures to maintain the tissues at the desired position.

Certain basic principles must be followed for successful suturing.

1. Use the least number of sutures necessary to accomplish the desired result.
2. Tension on the suture should be sufficient to hold the tissue in place, but not so great that tissue necrosis may result. In addition, too much tension may cause the suture to tear through the flap.
3. The sutures should be placed in keratinized tissue whenever possible.
4. Take an adequate "bite" of tissue with the suture needle to prevent the suture from tearing through the flap.

There is a variety of suture materials that may be used successfully. No suture material has all the desired characteristics. Monofilament and black silk sutures are used most often in periodontal surgery. Use the smallest size suture material that is compatible with the surgical procedure performed. Sterile (generally 0-4 or 0-5) prepackaged swaged ½ to ⅜ circle reverse cutting or tapered needles are recommended for most periodontal surgery.

There are numerous suturing techniques that are applicable to periodontal surgery. The four most common techniques are the interrupted suture, the sling suture, the continuous suture, and the vertical mattress suture.

1. *Interrupted suture.* This suture can be used for virtually all flap and graft surgery. It has its greatest application when both tissue margins require the same amount of tension, as in interproximal tissue approximation (Fig. 11–5).
2. *Sling suture.* The sling suture encircles the tooth and is used primarily when a flap has been raised on one side of the tooth and it is undesirable to tie to the opposite side. These sutures are often used as suspensory sutures to hold a flap coronally, such as the laterally positioned flap (Fig. 11–6*a* and *b*).
3. *Continuous suture.* This suture is

similar to the sling suture. It is used when numerous teeth are involved in the surgery, but a flap was elevated on only one side of the teeth. There is a variation, the double continuous suture, that may be used to suture flaps that have been elevated on both the facial and lingual surfaces of the teeth (Fig. 11–7 *a* and *b*).

4. *Mattress suture.* The mattress suture (vertical or horizontal) offers the advantage of keeping the suture material out from under the margin of the flap. This suture is often used for interproximal tissue approximation over bone grafts, and in excisional new attachment procedures, and for replaced flaps (Fig. 11–8 *a*, horizontal mattress; Fig. 11–8 *b*, vertical mattress).

Dressing

Purposes

Periodontal dressings are used after surgery for three reasons: to protect the wound area, to enhance patient comfort, and to help hold flaps in position. The two dressings most commonly used are zinc oxide-eugenol dressings and zinc oxide-noneugenol dressing. Currently, the noneugenol dressings are more popular. There are some clinicians who believe the use of periodontal dressing after flap surgery is not necessary.

A variety of zinc oxide-eugenol and zinc oxide-noneugenol periodontal dressing materials are available commercially. These materials should be prepared according to the manufacturer's directions. A lubricant should be placed on the fingers before handling the dressing. The dressing should be formed into small rolls approximately the same length as the surgical site. The material is adapted over the surgical area so that the apical one third of the clinical crown is covered, and it should be extended apically to ensure coverage of the surgical area without impinging on the mucobuccal fold or the floor of the mouth. A slightly dampened cotton tip applicator is used to apply gentle pressure to the dressing interproximally. Care should be taken to ensure that the dressing is not forced under the flaps. Use a *minimal* amount of dressing material to cover the surgical site adequately.

The initial dressing is left in place for about 1 week. When it is removed, the entire area is cleansed with warm water or diluted hydrogen peroxide. Any dressing fragments found embedded in soft tissue or in interproximal areas are removed. The tooth surfaces are carefully examined, and any accumulated plaque, debris, or remaining calculus or dressing material is removed coronal to the gingival margins by using an appropriate low abrasive paste. The patient is instructed in plaque control. The principal criteria for replacement of the dressing are the patient's comfort and the ability to remove plaque without damaging the healing tissue. Ideally, the patient should receive weekly recalls for polishing and plaque-control instruction during the first month(s) after surgery.

POST-SURGICAL CONSIDERATIONS

Postoperative Instructions

The patient should be provided with written postoperative instructions. The written instructions must be *carefully* reviewed with the patient before dismissal from the dental office.

Written instructions need not be elaborate and can be tailored to the individual. For example, a patient who has undergone surgery can be given the following instructions:

Postoperative Information

The following information has been prepared to help answer questions that

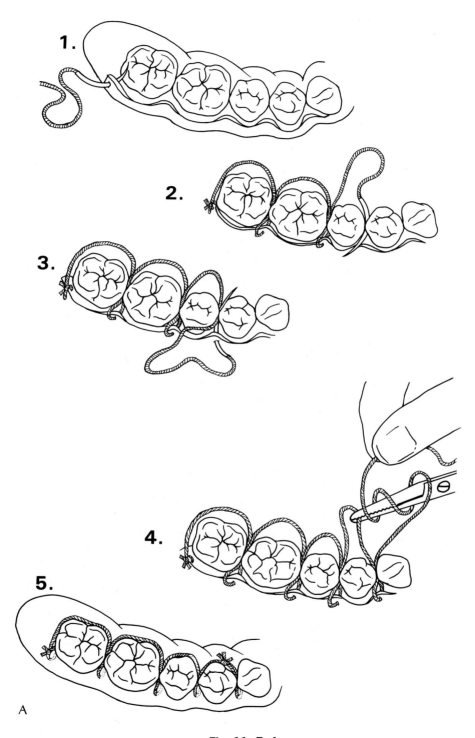

Fig. 11–7. A

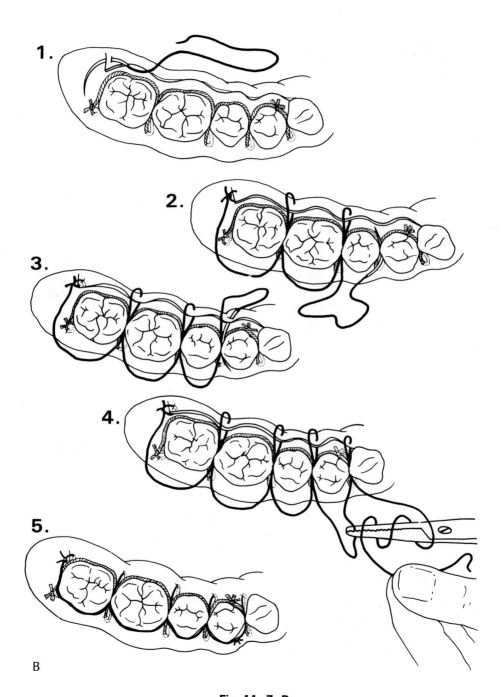

Fig. 11–7. B

B

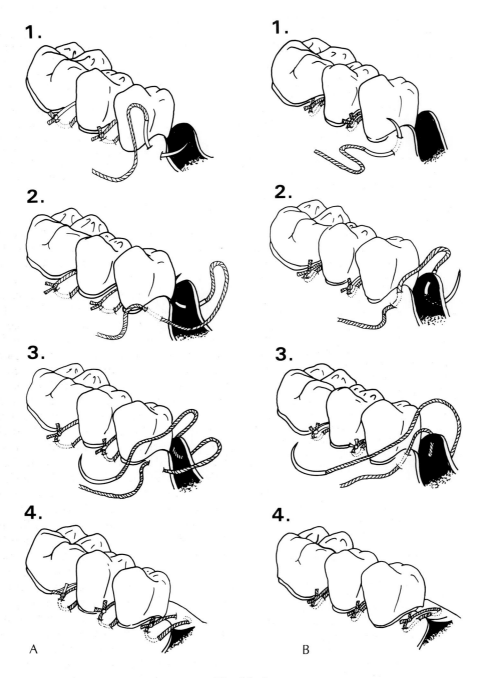

1.

2.

3.

4.

A   B

Fig. 11–8.

you may have after your periodontal (gum) surgery.

I. *Discomfort and Swelling.* Usually there is minimal discomfort or swelling after periodontal (gum) surgery. Should you become uncomfortable, take the analgesic tablets you have obtained by prescription. Be sure to follow exactly the instructions on the label on the bottle. Alcoholic beverages should not be consumed when taking analgesics. There are times that a recommendation will be made to use an icebag to control possible swelling. The icebag should be placed on the face, 15 minutes on, 15 minutes off, for the first hour.

II. *Bleeding.* Usually all bleeding has stopped by the time you leave the dental office. Do not be concerned if your saliva is a light pink color for a few hours after surgery. If you begin to bleed heavily, contact your dentist immediately. Do *not* suck liquid through a straw during the first 24 hours.

III. *Physical Activity.* It is recommended that you rest and curtail your physical activity the day of surgery. The day after surgery, you many resume your normal activities. It is recommended that you do not engage in strenuous physical activity during the first week after the surgery.

IV. *Nutrition.* Excellent nutrition is essential for proper healing. Do not utilize those areas where the surgery was performed to chew or bite until the areas have healed. Do not drink alcoholic beverages during the first 24 hours after surgery.

V. *Oral Hygiene.* The most important element required for good healing is meticulous plaque control. You may begin to brush your teeth the day of the surgery. The day after surgery you should thoroughly brush and floss all your teeth. If a dressing has been placed, you will be unable to floss this area.

VI. *Dressings.* Many times a pink-colored dressing will be placed over the surgical area. It is intended that the dressing remain in place for 1 week. It is of no concern if a few pieces of the dressing break off. However, if the dressing seems to be loose or has come off, contact this office immediately.

VII. *Antibiotics.* Antibiotics are not routinely given before or after periodontal surgery. If, however, antibiotics have been prescribed for you, it is essential that you take ALL the medication in accordance with the directions on the bottle.

VIII. *Other Medications.* Take any other medications as prescribed. Pay careful attention to the directions on the bottle. If you have any questions or any adverse reactions, contact the doctor immediately.

IX. You must return to this office in one week to have the sutures and/or the dressing removed. If you have any concerns regarding the surgery that has been performed, contact this office immediately (phone number _____).

Postoperative Problems

Bleeding and loose or lost dressings are infrequent problems after surgery, but they are the most common problems. When a patient returns to the dental office because of bleeding, the dressing should usually be removed entirely. The source of bleeding should be located by gently removing any clots that conceal it. Pressure applied to the site with gauze soaked in saline solution about 5 minutes usually stops the bleeding. If it does not, another 5-minute application is indicated. Frequently, injection of the bleeding site with an anesthetic containing 1:50,000 epinephrine will stop the bleeding. If the above procedures do not control the hemorrhage, oxidized cellulose (Surgicel) or microfibrillar collagen hemostat (Avitene) may be applied to the bleeding site. Uncontrolled bleeding may be an indication of a deficiency in bleeding or clotting mechanism, and an evaluation of these systems may be required, including questioning the patient about aspirin intake. If the problem is a loose dressing, the dressing should be entirely removed and a new dressing should be placed after cessation of any resultant bleeding.

Tense swelling, severe pain, obvious purulence, or fever and malaise indicate infection, which should be treated promptly and vigorously. Infection rarely follows careful periodontal surgery, but if it does, penicillin, erythromycin, or another appropriate antibiotic can be used effectively.

Postoperative root sensitivity may occur after dressings have been removed, and usually results from ineffective plaque control. Treatment of root sensitivity is discussed in Chapter 20. Because of greater emphasis on plaque control and on new attachment procedures rather than on resection, root sensitivity is not as common a complaint as in years past.

LIMITATIONS OF SURGERY

Surgery is not curative. It is a means of providing access to the deeper tissues and to the root surface, and of restoring missing parts of the periodontium. When surgery is performed for motivated, cooperative patients by skilled, knowledgeable practitioners, it is an important part of periodontal treatment.

CHAPTER 12

Management of Soft Tissue: Conservative New Attachment

POCKET ELIMINATION

The periodontal pocket is a space bounded by the tooth on one side and ulcerated epithelium lining the soft tissue wall on the other. Its base is on the coronal aspect of the epithelial attachment. The pocket can be eliminated by removing the tooth surface (extraction or root removal) or by altering the pocket walls.

There are four general approaches to management of the soft tissue wall and elimination of the space: 1) shrinkage of the soft tissue wall; 2) resection of the soft tissue wall; 3) new attachment of soft tissue wall to the tooth; and 4) movement of the soft tissue wall apically.

Shrinkage

Removal of plaque, calculus, and exposed cementum by scaling and root planing will reduce inflammation and effect shrinkage of the tissue. The amount of shrinkage can be quite traumatic. Many areas considered initially to require further treatment by surgery are later found to require no additional treatment.

Resection

Resection of the soft tissue wall is accomplished by gingivectomy, which is discussed in Chapter 13.

New Attachment

New attachment implies formation of new cementum, connective tissue fibers, and epithelial attachment on previously diseased root surfaces. In some cases, bone regeneration may occur. Many surgical procedures result in an attachment of tissue to tooth during healing, but this attachment is often at, or is apical to, the pre-existing level. To achieve *new* attachment at a more coronal level, certain procedures must be accomplished during surgery: 1) All pocket and attachment epithelium must be removed. 2) Cementum in the environment of the pocket must be detoxified. 3) Apposition of tissue to tooth surface must be as close as possible, facially, lingually, and proximally, with a minimal intervening blood clot. The smaller the clot, the more quickly granulation tissue cells can approach the tooth and produce the needed support elements. 4) Primary wound closure is ideal.

New attachment techniques that will be considered are: subgingival curettage and gingival flaps, such as the excisional new attachment procedure and the modified excisional new attachment procedure (Fig. 12–1*a–c*). Flap procedures (replaced flap and flap curettage) employed for the purpose of gaining new attachment of gingival tissues is discussed in Chapter 14.

SUBGINGIVAL CURETTAGE

Indications

The classic indications for subgingival curettage are the presence of shallow pockets and an adequate width and thickness of gingival tissue that is swollen, inflamed, and nonfibrotic.

Objective

The objective of this procedure is pocket elimination by shrinkage and new attachment.

Technique

The procedure is performed under local anesthesia. The objective is to detoxify the root surface, being careful to remove loosened calculus completely from the pocket (Fig. 12–1a) and then to peel out the epithelial lining and granulomatous tissue with a sharp curet. When hemostasis is achieved, sutures may be necessary to stabilize the tissue to the tooth. A periodontal dressing is used to cover the area.

Subgingival curettage with a curet is possibly talked about and written about more often than it is actually performed. First, it is a somewhat demanding tech-

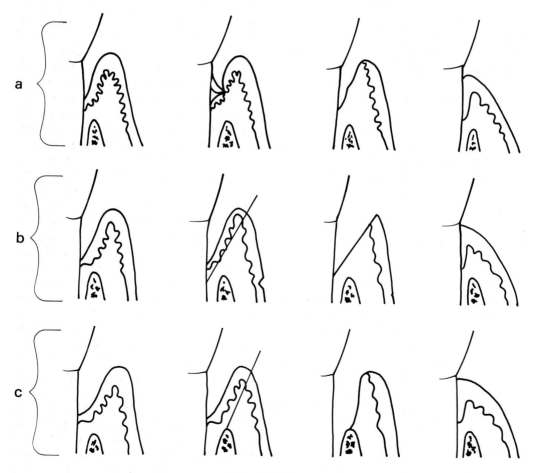

Fig. 12–1.

nical procedure, requiring sharp curets and great finesse. Second, it is a rather crude surgical procedure that macerates tissue, requiring further clean-up by phagocytic cells during healing. Third, root visualization is poor unless the pockets have been expanded by leaving some type of "packing" in them for a few days preoperatively.

It is hoped that a new attachment forms during healing. Although this may occur, the reduction in pocket depth is usually the result of the removal of tissue during curettage and shrinkage after healing. Deliberate subgingival curettage can sometimes be a useful technique in periodontal treatment. If shrinkage by resolution of inflammation is desired, however, it can be attained by removal of the etiologic agents. If diminution in bulk is desired, this result can be achieved by surgical procedures less traumatic and more predictable than the comparative blind scraping with a curet. Isolated pockets (e.g., a deep pocket on the palatal aspect of a maxillary canine), whether or not the tissue is fibrosed, may warrant an attempt at subgingival curettage. This procedure is especially helpful in the treatment of isolated pockets in the maintenance patient.

EXCISIONAL NEW ATTACHMENT PROCEDURE (ENAP)

The ENAP has been defined as a gingival flap. In essence, this procedure is subgingival curettage performed with a knife. The inner aspect (epithelium and some connective tissue) of the periodontal pocket is excised and the remaining gingival tissue is closely approximated against and between the teeth, providing the potential for formation of a new attachment during healing.

Indications

The ENAP is indicated: 1) in suprabony pockets of shallow moderate pocket depths that have an adequate zone of keratinized tissue; and 2) in the anterior region, where esthetics is a consideration.

Objective

The objective of ENAP is pocket reduction by establishing a new attachment to the tooth at a more coronal level. There is little question that some shrinkage occurs in this surgical procedure, but clinical studies also indicated a more coronal attachment of soft tissue.

Technique

Figures 12–1b to 12–4 illustrate the ENAP technique. Once the patient has established adequate plaque control and initial preparation is complete: 1) Anesthetize the area. 2) Measure pocket depth with a probe, and penetrate the gingival tissue at this distance with the probe (Fig. 12–2a). 3) Make an internally beveled incision with a surgical blade from the margin of the free gingiva apically to a point below the lowest point of the pocket (Fig. 12–1b). 4) Carry the incision interproximally on both the facial and lingual sides, attempting to retain as much interproximal tissue as possible (Fig. 12–3). The intention is to cut out the inner portion of the soft tissue wall of the pocket, all around the tooth. No attempt is made to elevate a flap. 5) Remove the excised tissue with a curet. 6) Carefully detoxify all cementum that has been exposed to the oral cavity to a smooth, hard consistency (Fig. 12–2c). Preserve all connective tissue fibers that remain attached to the root surface. 7) Rinse the area with sterile water or sterile normal saline solution, and examine the root surface to ensure no calculus remains and no large clots are present. 8) Approximate the wound edges. If the edges do not meet passively, contour the bone until good adaptation of the wound edges is achieved (Fig. 12–4). 9) Suture interproximally with interrupted or vertical mattress sutures. 10) Apply pressure for 2 to 3 minutes to the

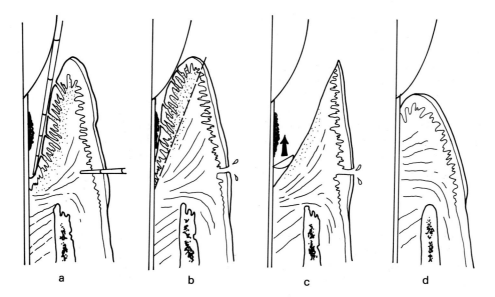

a   b   c   d

Fig. 12—2.

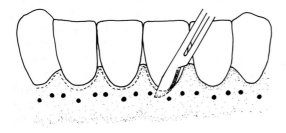

Fig. 12—3.

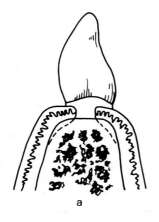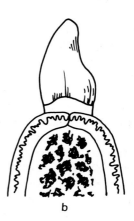

a   b

Fig. 12—4.

operative site from both facial and lingual aspects with saline-soaked gauze to permit only a small blood clot to form between the tissue and the tooth. 11) Place a periodontal dressing over the site without forcing the dressing between the tooth and the tissue. 12) Remove the sutures in 7 to 10 days and polish the area. Carefully review plaque control of the surgical area with the patient. Advise the patient to brush and to floss the area carefully and meticulously. A roll tooth-brushing technique and utilization of interproximal flossing to the gingival margin during the initial period will provide adequate plaque control without disrupting the healing of the gingival tissue to the tooth surface. Success is dependent on controlling plaque formation during the critical first 4 weeks of healing. 13) Do not probe for 3 months to permit complete attachment of connective tissue fibers.

The ENAP is a comparatively simple surgical procedure with the objective of reducing the pocket by establishing a new attachment at a more coronal level (Fig. 12–2d). Clinical experience has demonstrated the technique to be a predictable and effective method of eliminating suprabony pockets when care is exercised in case selection and execution of the procedure.

MODIFIED ENAP

The modified ENAP has also been defined as a gingival flap. In this variation, the primary modifications are: 1) The initial incision is directed toward the alveolar crest rather than toward the base of the periodontal pocket; 2) A secondary sulcular incision is made to the bone to facilitate removal of the connective tissue still attached to the tooth (Fig. 12–5).

The main advantages of the modified procedure when compared to the ENAP are the increased ease of performance resulting from directing the incision toward the alveolar crest instead of the base of

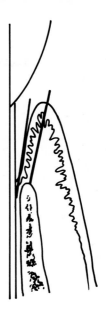

Fig. 12–5.

the pocket, greater access for root preparation due to additional tissue removal, and the potential for utilizing the healing capacity of the periodontal ligament. A potential disadvantage of this modification may be the removal of the intact attached connective tissue fibers (approximately 1 mm) coronal to the alveolar crest. The increased ease of soft tissue wall preparation, however, may make this more applicable to the majority of practitioners.

Clinical Application

Currently evidence does not provide specific indications for each of the gingival new attachment procedures. This determination is usually based on the clinical experiences and training of the clinician. A prerequisite common to all gingival new attachment procedures is the presence of an adequate amount, in width and thickness, of keratinized gingiva. The following general comments may be useful as a guide for selecting a surgical approach when new attachment and minimal post-surgical recession are the goals.

1. Scaling and root planing may be the

best technique for treating shallow lesions.

2. Meticulous attention to detail in performing the procedure is necessary to achieve a satisfactory result.

3. In the hands of a skilled clinician, subgingival curettage can be an effective technique for new attachment in isolated deeper pockets as well.

4. Curettage may be the treatment method used in compromise cases and for the active maintenance and retreatment of previously treated cases.

5. The ENAP and the modified procedure may be preferred in the management of suprabony pockets, particularly those in the maxillary anterior region.

6. Because no attempt is made to elevate the gingival tissue from the bone, post-surgical recession and trauma to the patient, as well as patient discomfort and root sensitivity, are minimized.

7. Clinical results indicate that pockets can be reduced or eliminated by gingival surgery techniques that seek new attachment of the soft tissue to the tooth.

8. Clinical new attachment is an achievable, predictable, and maintainable goal with any of the procedures described in this chapter, provided there is adequate long-term follow-up care.

CHAPTER 13

Management of Soft Tissue: Gingivoplasty and Gingivectomy

The chief purpose of gingivoplasty is the restoration of physiologic gingival contours that will help prevent recurrence of periodontal disease. The restoration of an esthetic appearance is also an important consideration. Gingivectomy is the excision of the gingival walls of a periodontal pocket; therefore, the purpose of gingivectomy is the elimination of a pocket. Both procedures should result in increased access for plaque control by the patient.

GINGIVOPLASTY

Indications

Gingivoplasty is usually indicated when physiologic contours are not present and the tissues are firm, fibrotic, and easily excised and contoured. This type of tissue most frequently results from chronic irritation.

Technique

Gingivoplasty entails the beveling of the gingival margin and/or interdental papillae with the creation of interdental spillways by blending the architecture of the interdental papillae with the interdental grooves (festooning). Usually, gingivoplasty is performed with a periodontal knife or coarse diamond stones.

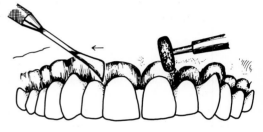

Fig. 13–1.

1. When a periodontal knife, such as Kirkland No. 15 or 16, is used, the tissue is excised to establish the basic contours. The knife is then used to scrape the tissue to achieve the final gingival architecture (Fig. 13–1).
2. Coarse diamond stones may also be used (Fig. 13–1). The stones may be of various shapes depending upon the need and preference of the clinician. A steady stream of sterile saline solution or sterile water must be used to prevent burning of the tissue and clogging of the stone. When stones are used, the soft tissue will often show minute shreds or tags, which can be removed with fine scissors or nippers.

After the gingiva has been contoured by either of the techniques described, a periodontal dressing is placed over the

109

area. The dressing is changed weekly until sufficient healing has occurred to permit plaque control by the patient. At each dressing change, the operator should gently remove any accumulated plaque and debris with floss or tape proximally, and with a curet. The teeth in the operative site should then be polished with a cup and low-abrasive polishing agent facially and lingually, avoiding damage to the healing tissue. At the time of final dressing removal, all teeth are polished again, and the patient is reinstructed in plaque-control procedures.

GINGIVECTOMY

Indications

This procedure may be indicated for elimination of periodontal pockets when excision of the pocket wall will not result in an inadequate zone of attached gingiva. Some examples of disease entities that usually can be treated by gingivectomy are:
1. Dilantin hyperplasia.
2. Chronic inflammatory hyperplasia.
3. Delayed passive eruption.
4. Hereditary fibromatosis.

Contraindications

Gingivectomy is not recommended in certain instances.
1. Where the pocket depths are at or are apical to the mucogingival junction.
2. Where the alveolar mucosa forms the soft tissue wall of the pocket.
3. When frenum and/or muscle attachments are in the area of surgery.
4. When treatment of infrabony defects is indicated.
5. When an esthetic deformity may result.

Technique
1. As a first step in gingivectomy, obtain satisfactory anesthesia by either the block or the infiltration technique.
2. Measure the pocket depths with a calibrated probe. These levels are marked by puncturing the outer wall of the gingival tissue with the probe to establish bleeding points. When the entire area has been ad-

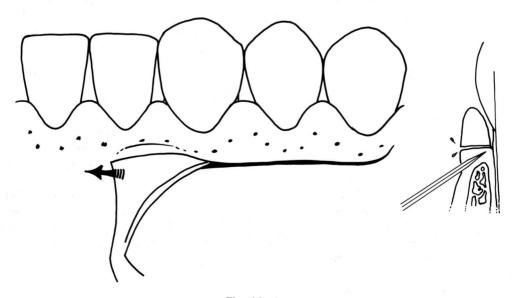

Fig. 13–2.

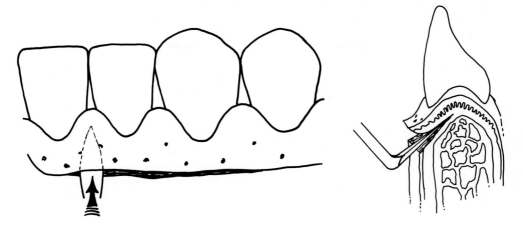

Fig. 13–3.

equately measured and marked, the bleeding points will outline the required incision.

3. Make the initial incision apical to the bleeding points with a broad-bladed knife such as Kirkland No. 15 or 16 (Fig. 13–2). The incision should be beveled to about a 45° angle to the root of the tooth and should end on the tooth at the depth of the pocket. Where the gingiva is thick, lengthen the bevel to eliminate a plateau or shoulder. Sometimes, access may be so limited or difficult that a proper bevel cannot be obtained with the initial incision. In this case, the bevel can be corrected later, either with a broad-bladed knife used as a scraper or with coarse abrasive rotary diamond stones.

4. Use narrow-bladed knives, such as the Orban Nos. 1 and 2, to excise the tissue interproximally (Fig. 13–3).

5. Remove the incised gingival tissue with curets (Fig. 13–4).

6. Remove accretions from the root surfaces by scaling and root planing. Removal of the soft tissue walls of periodontal pockets renders the

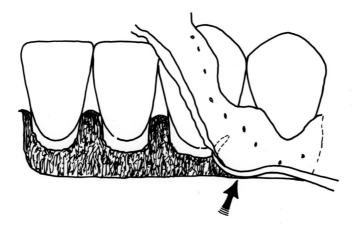

Fig. 13–4.

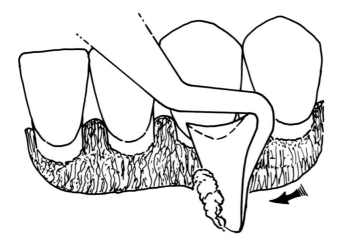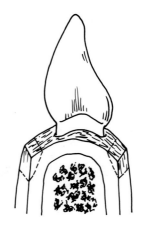

Fig. 13—5.

root surfaces more accessible and visible to the operator now than at any other time. Success or failure of the entire procedure depends on how well the operator performs root preparation.

7. Complete further contouring as needed by using coarse diamond stones or a broad-bladed knife to scrape the tissue (Fig. 13–5).

8. Remove tissue tags with scissors.

9. Flush the surgical site with sterile water or sterile saline solution to remove foreign particles.

10. Apply constant pressure against the wound for 2 to 3 minutes with cotton-free gauze sponges saturated with sterile water or sterile saline solution to stop bleeding.

11. Apply periodontal dressing by initially placing small, pointed sections of the dressing interproximally with a plastic instrument. Next, place longer strips on the facial, lingual, and palatal aspects and join them to the interproximal sections. Cover the entire wound area with the dressing, taking care not to let it interfere with occlusion or muscle attachments. A common error is to make the dressing too large.

12. Change dressing and debride the wound weekly until the tissues have healed sufficiently for the patient to accomplish plaque control. Remember, epithelium will cover a wound at the rate of 0.5 mm per day after an initial absence of mitotic epithelial activity 24 hours postoperatively.

13. After the dressing is removed, polish the teeth and instruct the patient in plaque control.

CHAPTER 14

Management of Soft Tissue: Flaps for Pocket Management

BASIC CONCEPTS AND CONSIDERATIONS

Objectives of Flaps

Generally, flap techniques are designed to accomplish one or more of the following.

1. Provide access for root preparation.
2. Eliminate pockets that extend to or beyond the mucogingival junction.
3. Preserve or create an adequate zone of attached gingiva.
4. Permit access to underlying bone for treatment of osseous defects.

Classification of Flaps

A flap is defined as that portion of the gingiva, alveolar mucosa, or periosteum that is elevated or dissected from the alveolar process and that retains its blood supply. Flaps may be classified on the basis of tissue components and positioning of these components at the completion of surgery. The following section is a classification and description of the more popular flap techniques for pocket management.

Flap Types

Full-Thickness Flap

The full-thickness (mucoperiosteal) flap is composed of mucosa, submucosa, and periosteum. It is prepared by bluntly dissecting soft tissue from the bone with a periosteal elevator. The technique is as follows.

1. Make a scalloped, internally beveled incision to the crest of the alveolar bone, preserving as much keratinized gingiva as possible. Scalpel blades Nos. 11, 12-b, 15, or 15c are commonly used to make this incision. The No. 11 or 15c blade in a modified handle works well on the lingual or palatal surfaces (Fig. 14–1a and b). The primary incision extends around the necks of the teeth and interproximally, to preserve the interproximal papillary tissue for primary wound closure.
2. Bluntly separate the tissue from the bone with a periosteal elevator to obtain sufficient access and flap mobility (Fig. 14–1c).
3. Make a sulcular incision around each tooth with the scalpel blade, Fedi chisels, or Ochsenbein chisels to sever the supracrestal gingival fibers from the tooth (Fig. 14–1d).
4. The scalpel blade or gingivectomy knives are used to sever the remaining collar of tissue by cutting horizontally at the crest of the bone (Fig. 14–1e).

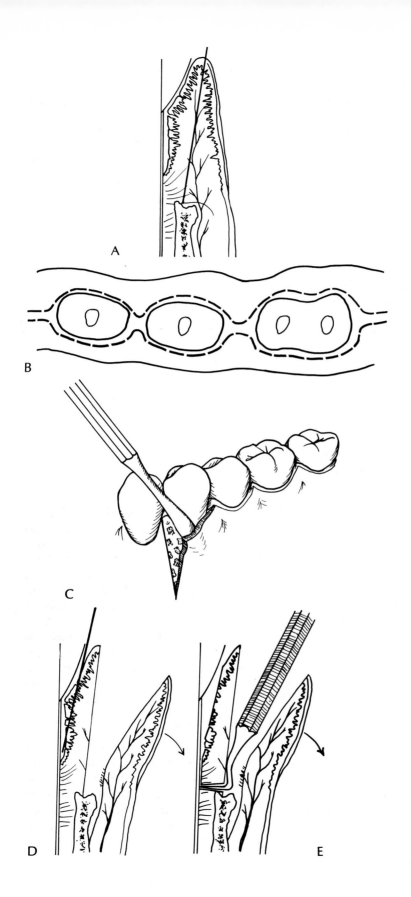

A

B

C

Fig. 14–1.

D

E

5. Remove the excised collar of tissue with a curet.
6. Root plane the granulomatous tissue from the osseous defects.
7. Root plane the involved root surfaces until smooth and hard. Remember connective tissue fibers attached to the root surfaces should be left attached. Only the root surfaces that had been exposed to the environment of the pocket need be treated. Citric acid (pH 1) applied for 3 minutes and rinsed thoroughly with sterile saline may be an aid to root detoxification.
8. Irrigate the surgical site and examine for any residual root accretions or tissue tags.
9. Treat bony defects by debridement, grafting, or osseous resection depending on the type of defect (see Chapter 16).
10. Depending on the surgical site and the surgical objective, the flap can be replaced by suturing near its original position or can be apically positioned.
11. Apply firm but gentle pressure for 2 to 3 minutes on the facial and lingual flaps with gauze moistened in sterile saline solution.
12. Some clinicians apply Orabase or another ointment to prevent wedging of dressing beneath the flap and to prevent the dressing from binding to the sutures.
13. Remove dressing and sutures after 7 to 10 days. Carefully debride and polish the area. Instruct the patient in proper plaque control.

Vertical Relaxing Incisions

These incisions may be employed on the facial surface when access and visibility are limited. They should be made at line angles to preserve the interdental papillae for suturing and to prevent necrosis of the wound edge (Fig. 14–2a). Under no circumstances should vertical incisions

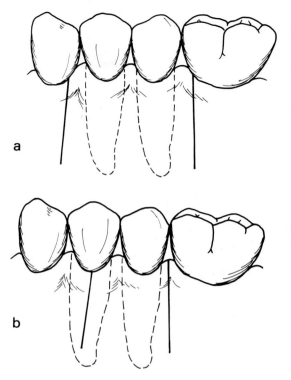

Fig. 14–2.

be made over the midfacial (radicular) surface of roots (Fig. 14–2b). Vertical relaxing incisions should not be performed indiscriminately. There are certain disadvantages associated with them, such as: 1) a greater opportunity for undesirable flap displacement; and 2) an increase in the likelihood of postoperative swelling, bleeding and patient discomfort. Also, vertical incisions are not recommended on most areas of the palate and the mandibular lingual surface because of surgical and postoperative complications of bleeding, nerve damage, and infection.

Partial-Thickness Flap

The partial-thickness (mucosal) flap is composed of mucosa only, or mucosa and submucosa. It is prepared by sharp dissection close to the bone with the intent of leaving some connective tissue attached to and covering the bone. The technique is as follows:

1. Make a scalloped, internally beveled incision from the surface of the tissue to the crest of the alveolar process, preserving as much tissue as possible (Fig. 14–3a). Scalpel blades Nos. 11, 12-b, 15, or 15c are commonly used.
2. A second incision is directed apically around the necks of the teeth to sever the supracrestal gingival fibers from the tooth (Fig. 14–3a).
3. Remove the excised collar of tissue with a curet.
4. Make an incision with a scalpel parallel to and close to the bone, leaving about a 0.5 to 1.0 mm thickness of soft tissue attached to bone (Fig. 14–3b). The flap is easily dissected if light tension is placed on the coronal portion of the flap. This tension can be accomplished by placing a suture or small tissue hook through the flap or by having the surgical assistant aid in retraction (Fig. 14–3b). Vertical relaxing incisions can be made as needed.
5. Thoroughly scale and plane the previously exposed roots. Care is taken not to remove connective tissue fibers attached to the roots.
6. Depending on the surgical site and the surgical objective, the flap is either replaced, using appropriate suturing techniques, or is apically positioned (Fig. 14–3c).
7. Apply firm but gentle pressure for 2 or 3 minutes on the facial and lingual flaps with gauze moistened in sterile saline solution.
8. Some clinicians apply Orabase or another ointment to prevent wedging of dressing beneath the flap and binding of the dressing to the sutures.

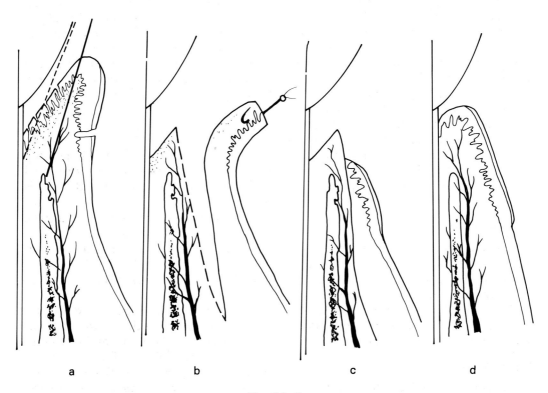

a   b   c   d

Fig. 14–3.

9. Remove dressing and sutures after 7 to 10 days and carefully polish the area. Instruct the patient in plaque control. Healing will generally occur as seen in Figure 14–3d.

Full-Thickness versus Partial Thickness Flaps

There are differences of opinion regarding the routine use of either a partial-thickness or a full-thickness flap. Some clinicians believe that bone loss is less likely to be permanent if partial-thickness flaps are used. Others have shown that full-thickness flaps actually result in less bone loss. Advocates of full-thickness flaps will point out that there is greater likelihood of necrosis of wound edges of the partial-thickness flap due to reduced blood supply. Also, surgical perforation is more likely in the partial-thickness flap. These complications could result in loss of tissue and delayed healing.

In actual practice, partial-thickness flaps are difficult to perform and true indications for their use are infrequent. Although this technique may seem to be indicated in areas of thin gingival and/or mucosal tissue (e.g., prominent roots), the thinness of the tissue presents technical problems at incision and there is the possibility that the blood supply will be compromised. A preferable technique may be to perform a full-thickness flap, but not to instrument the connective tissue on the root surface.

Flap Placement

The flap procedures most frequently utilized in periodontal surgery for pocket management are the replaced flap and the apically positioned flap. Facial and lingual aspects of a surgical site may involve any combination of the two types of flaps, depending on therapeutic goals.

Replaced Flap

Indications. A replaced flap (also called repositioned flap and modified Widman flap) is one that is repositioned in or near its original position (Fig. 14–4a). It is used to:

1. Gain access to underlying bone and root surfaces.
2. Reduce pockets by establishing a new epithelial and/or connective tissue attachment at a more coronal level.
3. Achieve primary closure during osseous regeneration procedures.

The replaced flap is contraindicated if there is an inadequate zone of keratinized gingiva. In this instance, a technique such as the apically positioned flap is indicated, not only to increase the width of gingiva but also to dissipate the pull of the connective tissue and muscle fibers.

Technique. In the replaced flap procedure, a full-thickness flap is usually employed for access to the diseased roots and alveolar bone. At the completion of root preparation and osseous treatment, the flaps are replaced near their original position and are sutured (interrupted or vertical mattress) interproximally. Every attempt must be made to approximate wound edges and to obtain primary wound closure, particularly interdentally.

Apically Positioned Flap

Indications. An apically positioned flap is one that is placed apical to its original position at the end of the procedure. It is used to:

1. Eliminate pockets by positioning the gingival tissue apically.
2. Increase the zone of attached gingiva.
3. Expose additional root structure for restorative dentistry.

The latter two indications are accomplished by moving existing mature gingiva apically on the tooth and/or the alveolar process. Collagen fibers from the periodontal ligament and from the granulation tissue will form coronal to the margin of the apically positioned gingiva.

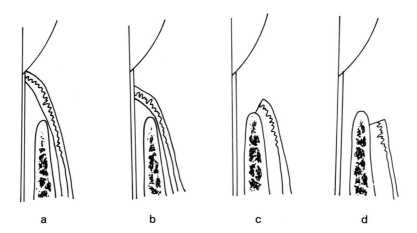

a   b   c   d

Fig. 14–4.

When mature, this tissue will function as additional attached gingiva.

The final position of the flap margin may vary according to clinical conditions and the desired results of surgery. Flaps may be moved apically so that the margin is positioned:

1. On the tooth root within 2 mm of the alveolar crest (APF-T) (Fig. 14–4*b*).
2. At the alveolar crest (APF-C) (Fig. 14–4*c*).
3. Apical to the alveolar crest (subcrestal) (APF-SC) (Fig. 14–4*d*).

Technique. The apically positioned flap procedure may involve the use of either a full-thickness or partial-thickness flap (Figs. 14–1 and 14–3). The following technique modifications/suggestions should be considered.

1. Because the interproximal apposition of wound edges is not a surgical goal, it is not critical to retain all of the interproximal tissue. A scalloped incision is generally preferable to a straight line incision, however, to retain a maximal amount of keratinized gingiva on the wound edge.
2. Reflect a full- or partial-thickness flap. It is common to begin by performing a partial-thickness flap in the gingiva and then to change to a full-thickness flap in the mucosa to achieve flap mobility and to preserve the blood supply.
3. On the palate, the bound masticatory mucosa does not allow the physical movement of the tissue. Any apical displacement of the margin must be accomplished by surgical reduction. The initial incision is made somewhat apical to the free gingival margin and is aimed at a point slightly apical to the alveolar crest. The exact position of this incision is based on the level of the palatal osseous tissues and the shape of the palatal vault (the shallower the palatal vault, the closer to the gingival margin the incision needs to be made). This type of incision results in a wedge of tissue (secondary flap) remaining between the outer (primary) flap and the tooth. The removal of this wedge of tissue with curets or hoes and the position of the initial incision determines the marginal height of the palatal tissues post surgically.
4. During root preparation, acid or other chemical root treatment is not indicated in apically positioned flap procedures. Care should be taken not to over-instrument the root sur-

face that will be coronal to the flap margin (to reduce post-surgical sensitivity).

5. Suture the flap margin so that it rests at or near the crest of the alveolar process (APF-T, APF-C, APF-SC). The most common error in suturing is to suture too tightly, pulling the flap coronally and defeating the purpose of the procedure.

CHAPTER 15

Management of Soft Tissue: Mucogingival Procedures

MUCOGINGIVAL CORRECTIVE SURGERY

Indications

Gingival atrophy and recession are important abnormalities of the mucogingival complex. Areas of recession may be the result of problems with the frenum and attached gingiva. Exposed root surfaces associated with recession may be unesthetic and painful. The determination and correction of etiologic factors (such as prominent tooth position, frena, tooth-brushing technique, restoration margins or contours, and factitious habits) are important in overall treatment success.

Objectives
1. Establish an adequate width or thickness of keratinized and attached gingiva.
2. Eliminate pull on the free gingival margin by freni or muscle attachments.
3. Correct gingival clefts or recession.
4. Establish new gingival attachment at a more coronal level.

Techniques

Mucogingival corrective procedures involve pedicle flap techniques and/or free soft tissue grafts. Pedicle flap procedures include the laterally positioned flap, the coronally positioned flap, and on occasion, the apically positioned flap. Free soft tissue grafts are usually autogenous (free gingival grafts). Recently, allogeneic materials such as freeze-dried skin and freeze-dried dura mater have been utilized in these gingival addition procedures.

Laterally Positioned Flap

This flap is used to move gingiva from an adjacent tooth or edentulous area to a prepared recipient site. This procedure requires that only one or two teeth need therapy and that sufficient width and thickness of donor tissue is available in adjacent areas. Also, adequate vestibular depth is necessary for one to perform a laterally positioned flap correctly. When adjacent tooth sites are to be used as donor areas, care must be exercised that the donor gingival tissue is not inflamed and is thick, wide, and keratinized. There should be no underlying bony fenestrations or dehiscences.

Indications. The laterally positioned flap is used to:
1. Increase the zone of attached gingiva.
2. Cover isolated areas of recession

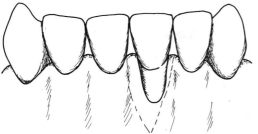

Fig. 15–1.

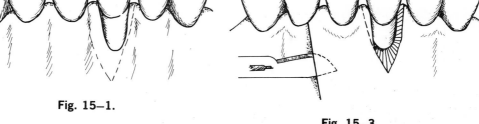

Fig. 15–3.

where the adjacent proximal gingival height is more coronal.

This procedure can also increase the zone of attached gingiva and cover root surfaces exposed as a result of recession. Either a full- or a partial-thickness flap can be utilized. Both types of flaps result in satisfactory clinical healing, but studies of root coverage suggest that full-thickness, laterally positioned flaps result in more connective tissue attachment than do partial-thickness, laterally positioned flaps. Partial-thickness flaps may be indicated when protection of the donor area (especially radicular surfaces) against bone loss is desired. Clinical root coverage of about 65% of the original recession area can be routinely expected. Similarly, about 1 mm of recession at the donor site usually occurs.

Technique

1. Make a V-shaped incision with a No. 15 blade and create a beveled wound edge around the recipient site (Figs.

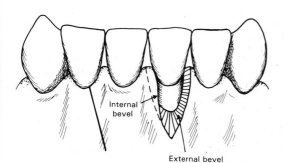

Fig. 15–2.

15–1 and 15–2). The wound edge to be sutured must be over bone.

2. Remove the incised tissue with a curet, and root plane the cementum until it is smooth and hard. The application of citric acid or other chemical root treatment may enhance the potential for a new connective tissue attachment.

3. Make a vertical incision at a distance of at least one and a half times the measurement of the recipient site. This incision should be angled slightly toward the recipient site (Fig. 15–2).

4. Perform either a full-thickness or partial-thickness dissection (Fig. 15–3) to free the donor flap tissue from its bed, being careful to maintain its base and blood supply. A useful modification is to perform a partial-thickness dissection in the gingiva and to shift to a full-thickness dissection in the mucosal region. Enough vestibular depth and mobility of the donor pedicle must be present to allow the unrestrained, relaxed positioning of the flap at the recipient site.

5. Position the flap at the recipient site to cover the defect completely. If there is tension on the flap as the lip or cheek is extended, further dissection and elevation at the base may be performed (Fig. 15–4).

6. Suture the flap to ensure coverage

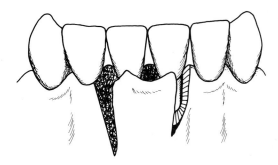

Fig. 15—4.

of the denuded root surface as shown in Figure 15–5. Place interrupted sutures (5-0 is preferred), beginning apically and working coronally. No more than two or three sutures are usually necessary. A sling suture is carried around the tooth and is tied facially to prevent the graft from slipping apically. Particular attention must be paid to the suturing of the apical area to immobilize the entire length of the flap to the bed.

7. Apply gentle but firm pressure to the flap for 2 to 3 minutes with cotton-free gauze moistened with sterile saline solution.

8. Cover the surgical site with an appropriate dressing to protect the flap from displacement. The dressing must not displace the flap or impinge on its base. An improperly placed dressing may impede the blood supply to the coronal part of

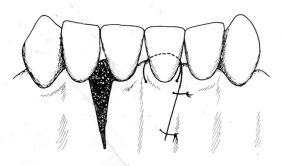

Fig. 15—5.

the flap and result in necrosis and failure.

9. Remove the dressing and sutures after 7 to 10 days, polish the area, and instruct the patient in plaque control. The area should not be probed for 3 months.

When properly performed, the laterally positioned flap is a predictable surgical procedure for increasing the zone of attached gingiva and/or repair of gingival clefts when there is sufficient width of keratinized gingiva at the donor site.

Double Papillae Flap

Indications. The double papillae flap is a modification of the laterally positioned flap. It can be used to repair gingival clefts when there is an adequate amount of healthy interproximal tissue adjacent to the recipient site and minimal keratinized gingiva over the radicular surfaces. Clinical situations favoring this procedure are few, because many recession areas are too wide for the papillae. In practice, many clinicians have had limited success with the double papillae flap.

Hattler Procedure

A variation of the laterally positioned flap in which the papillae are used as donor tissue in combination with an apically positioned flap is the Hattler procedure. This procedure is accomplished as part of pocket reduction therapy, wherein the entire flap is positioned apically and one-half tooth width mesially or distally so that the papillae rest on the midradicular surface of the teeth at or just coronal to the alveolar bone crest (Fig. 15–6). Since the papillae usually are 3 to 4 mm in length, this amount of keratinized gingiva is retained over the roots, and new attached gingiva and papillae will regenerate in the interproximal areas during healing. Generally, these interproximal areas heal without any residual bone or attachment loss. Surgically, some tissue must be removed from the flap

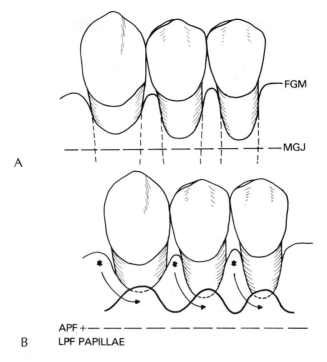

Fig. 15–6.

edge in the direction of movement so as not to overlap tissue surfaces, but the other steps are the same as those for laterally positioned and apically positioned flaps.

Free Gingival Graft (Free Soft Tissue Autograft)

Indications. The free soft tissue autograft is an extremely versatile and highly predictable technique. It is used to:

1. Increase the zone of attached gingiva.
2. Eliminate aberrant frena or muscle attachments.
3. Deepen the vestibule.
4. Repair gingival clefts.

Wound healing studies have demonstrated the effectiveness of the technique in the treatment of the first three aforementioned problems. These same studies, however, indicate that the free gingival graft can also repair narrow clefts, but would not adequately bridge deep, wide gingival clefts.

Technique

1. Make an internally beveled incision, using a No. 15 blade, 1 to 2 mm coronal to the mucogingival junction. This action may result in resection of the collar of gingival tissue (Figs. 15–7a and b).

2. Dissect the tissue close to the bone, leaving a thin connective tissue bed attached to bone. Extend the incision to include the involved teeth. Prepare the bed by removing excess connective tissue with iris scissors or tissue nippers. All muscle fibers must be removed (Figs. 15–7a and b; 15–8a and b; 15–9). Exposure of bone does not jeopardize the results.

3. Make a periosteal fenestration by exposing a small horizontal strip of bone near the apical border of the recipient site (Fig. 15–8b). The mucosal flap on the lip or cheek side

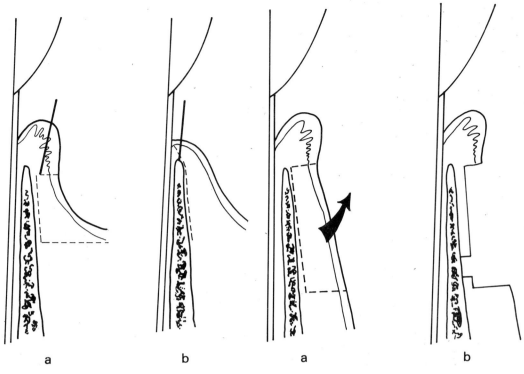

a   b

Fig. 15–7.

Fig. 15–8.

a   b

may be sutured to the reflected periosteum apical to the fenestration with small resorbable sutures.

4. Prepare a template of the recipient site by using the wrapper of the sterile surgical blade.

5. Take the template to the donor site (edentulous ridge or hard palate) and superficially outline with a blade. If the palate is used, care must be taken to avoid incorporating rugae in the graft or encroaching on the major palatal vessels.

6. Remove the donor tissue with a No. 15 blade or one of the special instruments designed to remove thin sections of tissue. The graft should be between 1.0 and 1.5 mm in thickness and should be wide enough to cover the recipient site. Achieve hemostasis of the donor site wound.

7. If the donor tissue is removed from the palate, all glandular tissue and

fat must be removed from the inner surface with iris scissors, or it will act as a barrier to the development of new circulation.

8. Rinse the undersurface of the graft and the recipient site with sterile saline solution to remove clots. Clot

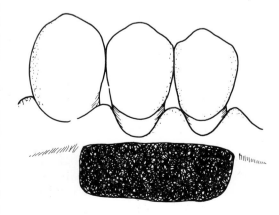

Fig. 15–9.

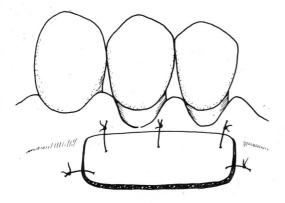

Fig. 15—10.

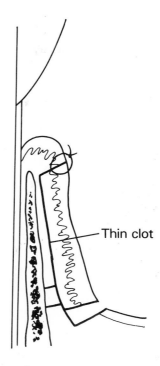

—Thin clot

Fig. 15—11.

formation will prevent initial nutrition of the graft by diffusion and will result in necrosis of the graft before revascularization can occur.

9. Suture the graft at the coronal margin to ensure immobilization (Fig. 15–10). Lateral and apical sutures may be used as desired to help stretch the graft slightly.

10. Apply gentle but firm pressure for 2 to 3 minutes with gauze moistened with sterile saline solution to assist in initial fibrin clot formation and effective union between the graft and the recipient site (Fig. 15–11).

11. Apply an appropriate protective dressing to the surgical site, being careful not to displace the graft.

12. Remove the dressing and sutures after 7 to 10 days, polish the area, and instruct the patient in plaque control. Caution the patient against disturbing the graft until clinical healing is complete. The area should not be probed for 3 months.

Healing of the recipient site is usually uneventful. A white, sloughing epithelial layer is present after 1 week and the graft is essentially united to the bed. Healing of the palatal donor site is usually more of a problem for the patient as the large denuded area slowly granulates and epithelializes. Dressing retention is difficult in the palate and many clinicians fabricate an acrylic stent to protect the area during healing.

A progressive coronal shift of the gingival tissue once an adequate band of attached gingiva has been established is common. This phenomenon is called creeping attachment and may result in complete or partial coverage of an exposed root surface.

Soft Tissue Allografts

A recent modification of the free gingival graft procedure is the use of allogeneic freeze-dried skin or freeze-dried dura mater obtained from a tissue bank as the donor material. The use of freeze-dried allogeneic material eliminates the need for a donor site and provides an abundant amount of tissue for multiple or extensive augmentation sites. The surgical principles of recipient site preparation are similar, but a periosteal bed is

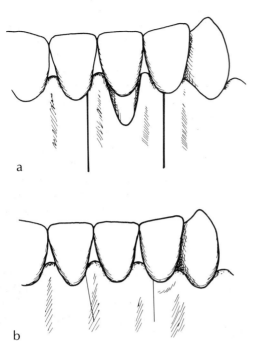

Fig. 15–12.

necessary; no studies of the use of freeze-dried materials on bare bone have been performed. The surgical sites heal with a gingival-type tissue and are usually more esthetic than some free gingival graft procedures. Freeze-dried skin allografts have also been used in combination with apically positioned flaps to cover the crestal alveolar bone and to provide a greater zone of keratinized gingiva.

Coronally Positioned Flaps

Another treatment alternative to correct areas of recession is the coronally positioned flap. This procedure is often preceded by a free gingival graft to increase the amount of gingival-type tissue available at the local site. Clinical evaluation demonstrates a rate of successful root coverage similar to that for laterally positioned flaps (Figs. 15–12a and b).

As usually performed, an initial surgical procedure, consisting of a free gin-gival graft or freeze-dried skin allograft, is performed apical to the area of recession and is allowed to heal for 6 to 8 weeks. Then, a full-thickness flap is reflected, with the use of vertical incisions at its lateral boundaries, to release the tissue and to allow it to be positioned and secured at a more coronal level. Thorough root planing and/or odontoplasty and/or citric acid may be used to prepare the root. Sutures, pressure, and dressing are used as in the other mucogingival procedures.

Combination Procedures

Many times these basic mucogingival procedures are performed in combination. A free gingival graft may be used to protect the donor site of a laterally positioned flap when the latter is indicated for root coverage. Free gingival grafts may be followed by a coronally positioned flap. Bone graft areas may be covered by free gingival grafts or freeze-dried skin allografts. The goals of treatment remain the same, but surgery is becoming more sophisticated in its accomplishments.

Other Considerations in Root Coverage

Two other factors that may influence the result of mucogingival procedures should be mentioned, and both relate primarily to root coverage attempts. The first involves the treatment of endodontically treated teeth. Conflicting reports and clinical impressions abound, but several research reports seem to indicate that root coverage attempts are as successful on endodontically treated teeth as on vital teeth.

Another factor influencing the success of root coverage is root preparation. Generally, cementum and dentin exposed to the oral cavity absorb endotoxins and other substances that have an adverse influence on fibroblasts and epithelial cells. As a general rule, aggressive scaling and root planing (and at times odontoplasty of the root) are recommended to remove enough root structure to eliminate these toxic substances, as well as to reduce the prominence of the root. Chemical root preparation agents, such as citric acid, may improve the predictability and degree of success.

MANAGEMENT OF OTHER SOFT TISSUE PROBLEMS

Aberrant Frena (Frenectomy)

Aberrant frena can be treated by incising the frenum at its insertion with or without placement of a free soft tissue graft. Occasionally a frenum, especially a maxillary labial or mandibular lingual frenum, is so large that it should be totally excised and the wound should be sutured. This procedure is termed a frenectomy. The techniqe for frenectomy is as follows.

1. Grasp the frenum with a slightly curved hemostat at its base. Cut the tissue with scissors above the hemostat and then below it, until the hemostat is free (Fig. 15–13a and b).

2. Use the scissors to remove any dense fibers that may be observed in the wound (Fig. 15–13c). Extend the lip and check to determine if there is still pull on the periosteum.

3. Suture the edges of the diamond-shaped wound together (Fig. 15–13d) to reduce postoperative discomfort and to promote healing.

4. Remove sutures after 7 to 10 days.

Shallow Vestibule (Vestibuloplasty)

A facial or labial vestibule that is too shallow for placement of a removable prosthetic appliance may be deepened by a free soft tissue gingival graft or an apically positioned flap.

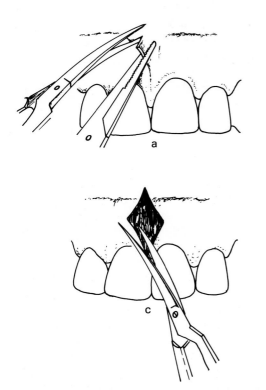

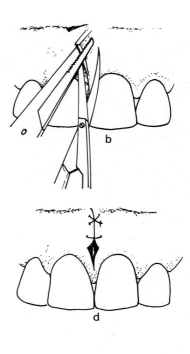

Fig. 15–13.

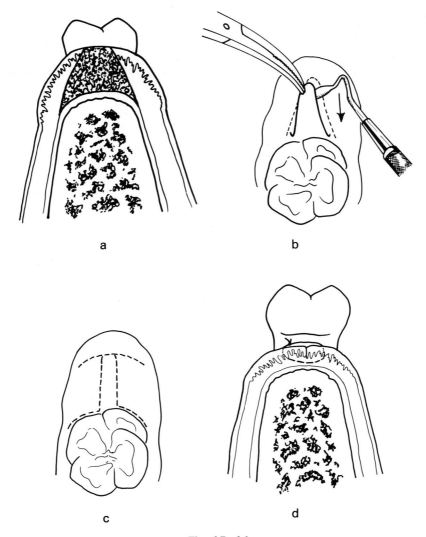

a   b

c   d

Fig. 15–14.

Deep Pocket Retromolar Area (Distal Wedge Procedure)

A deep pocket in the retromolar area may be corrected by a distal wedge or distal box procedure. The technique is as follows.

1. Use an undermining incision to prepare a partial-thickness flap on the facial and lingual surfaces of the retromolar area, as shown in Figure 15–14a, with a No. 12-b blade. If desired, parallel undermining facial and lingual incisions may be used, followed by a connecting incision at the distal aspect of the retromolar area; this results in a rectangular box rather than a wedge (Fig. 15–14c).

2. Grasp the wedge of tissue at the distal edge with a curved hemostat and remove it with an Orban knife (Fig. 15–14b).

3. Scale and root plane the distal surface of the molar.

4. Perform osseous surgery, if indicated. The distal surface of the second molar is a common area for a deep osseous defect, which may respond to bone-grafting procedures.

5. Approximate the wound edges and suture with interrupted sutures (Fig. 15–14*d*.).
6. Protect this area for 7 to 10 days with a periodontal dressing.

CHAPTER 16

Management of Osseous Defects: Osseous Resective Surgery

INTRODUCTION TO OSSEOUS SURGERY

An osseous defect is a concavity or deformity in the alveolar bone involving one or more teeth. Osseous surgery is the general term for all procedures designed to modify and reshape defects and deformities in the bone surrounding the teeth.

Diagnosis

A rational approach to osseous surgery must be based on the accurate diagnosis and morphologic classification of existing defects. It is important that the therapist determine the morphology of an osseous defect as accurately as possible. It is unfortunate that most of the methods for diagnosing osseous defects record the topography in a single plane in one spatial dimension. Routine probing will supply the linear measurement of probing depth. Radiopaque materials, such as Hirschfeld points and silver points, will disclose depth and contour of the pocket with respect to the bony outline (Fig. 16–1).

If local anesthesia is used, one can "sound" (probe both vertically and horizontally through the gingiva with a sharp instrument) to help determine the location and the number of osseous walls. The three-dimensional morphology of a defect, however, cannot usually be determined until the defect is visualized at the time of surgery.

Classification

Periodontal pockets with their base apical to the crest of the alveolar bone are called infrabony pockets. For these pockets to occur, there must be bone loss apical to the crest of the alveolar bone. The resultant bony defect is referred to as an infrabony defect (infrabony = below the bone). These infrabony defects can be classified according to the number of *remaining* osseous walls and by their morphology.

Three-Wall Defect

The three-wall infrabony defect occurs most frequently in the interdental region. The remaining walls are the facial, the lingual, and the proximal bone (Fig. 16–2). This defect is also referred to as an intrabony defect (intrabony = within the bone). A three-wall defect may also occur as a trough-like defect on the facial or lingual aspect. Occasionally, a three-wall defect may wrap around the tooth, involving two or more contiguous root surfaces (Fig. 16–3). These are referred to as circumferential defects. In addi-

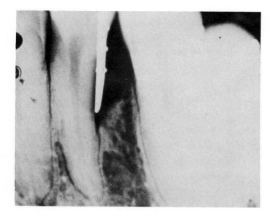

Fig. 16—1.

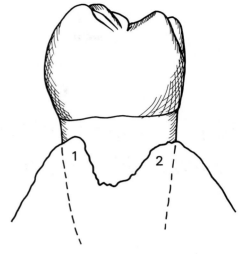

Fig. 16—4.

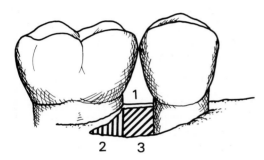

Fig. 16—2.

tion to designation by the number of remaining walls, the three-wall defect is described as narrow, wide-mouthed, shallow, or deep, depending on its dimensions.

Two-Wall Defect

The most prevalent osseous defect is the two-wall defect, referred to as a crater (Fig. 16—4). It is found interdentally and has a facial and a lingual wall. A two-wall defect can also occur when facial and proximal walls remain (Fig. 16—5).

One-Wall Defect

The one-wall defect usually occurs interdentally; if the remaining wall is the

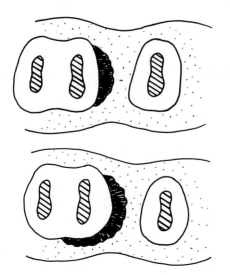

Fig. 16—3.

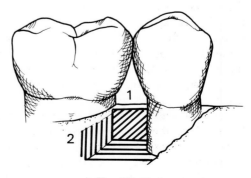

Fig. 16—5.

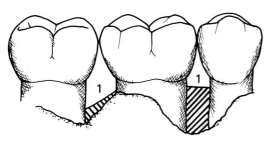

Fig. 16–6.

proximal wall, the defect is referred to as a hemiseptum. The remaining osseous wall may be on the facial or the lingual side (Fig. 16–6).

Combination

Many osseous lesions occur as some combinations of the one-, two-, and/or three-wall bony defects (Fig. 16–7). The depth, width, topography, and number of remaining osseous walls, and the configuration of the adjacent root surfaces are all important in determining the therapeutic approach.

Objectives

There are four basic objectives to be accomplished with osseous surgery:
1. To create contours that permit patients to accomplish effective plaque control.
2. To create contours that will parallel the contours of the gingival tissue after healing.
3. To permit primary wound closure.

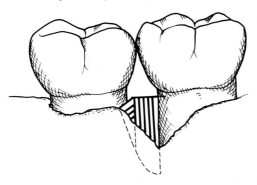

Fig. 16–7.

4. To expose additional clinical crown for proper construction of restorations (crown lengthening).

MANAGEMENT OF OSSEOUS DEFECTS

The therapist has five basic choices for resolving osseous defects.
1. Eliminate the defect by removing or recontouring nonsupporting bone (osteoplasty) or by removing tooth-supporting bone (ostectomy). Together, this procedure is referred to as osseous resective surgery.
2. Induce or promote regrowth and regeneration of bone. These regenerative techniques most often include bone grafts (see Chapter 17).
3. Amputate a root, in cases of interradicular involvement, or divide the tooth into two parts to eliminate the defect. These procedures also involve some bone recontouring (osseous resective surgery) to correct the bony defect adequately (see Chapter 18).
4. *Attempt* maintenance of the pocket and osseous defect by frequent scaling, root planing, topical antimicrobials, plaque control, or a combinations of these factors (see Chapter 19).
5. Extract the tooth.

Of these five methods of management of osseous defects, only osseous resective surgery will be discussed in this chapter.

Gingival Behavior

Before osseous resective surgery is performed, it is important to understand the normal relationship of gingiva to the tooth and underlying bone. It is also important to understand how gingiva behaves during healing after periodontal surgery.

In health, there is a somewhat constant relationship of the gingiva to the tooth. There is normally 1 mm of connective tissue attachment to the root. There is normally 1 mm of junctional epithelium along the tooth. Lastly, there is approximately a 1-mm space between the gingiva and the tooth called the sulcus. This easily remembered 1 mm:1 mm:1 mm relationship is referred to as the biologic width (Fig. 16–8).

Also observed in health are physiologic contours of the gingiva consisting of facial and lingual scalloping and interdental papillae. The degree of scalloping and papilla height varies in different places in the mouth. There are, however, biologic rules that can be used to determine normal physiologic contours. Scalloping tends to parallel the cementoenamel junction. More significant is the gingival relationship to the convexity of the root surface and the tooth position in the alveolar bone. The more convex anterior teeth have a greater degree of gingival scalloping than posterior teeth (Fig. 16–9). Gingiva on a prominent root in the arch has more scalloping than the gingiva on a normally positioned root. Teeth in close proximity have long, narrow papillae and therefore have greater scalloping than teeth with wide interdental areas. After periodontal surgery, the gingiva heal according to these anatomic concepts. Gingiva is always scalloped to some degree with greater scalloping on prominent convex roots. Posterior teeth, which before

surgery had flat gingival scalloping on a single root trunk, will often have a double, heavy scalloping on the two, now prominent facial roots.

After periodontal surgery, the gingiva also attempts to re-establish its biological width. If the bony contours are parallel to the final healed contours of the gingiva, the equal dimensions of the biologic width will be re-established. If the bony contours are not parallel to the final healed gingival contours, one of the dimensions of the biologic width will predominate. Although it is possible to achieve longer connective tissue and junctional epithelium, it is unlikely, especially in posterior areas. The sulcus, therefore, is the dimension that is most apt to increase in length. A deepened sulcus is difficult for the patient to keep clean. Therefore, periodontal disease tends to recur at these sites, resulting in recurrent periodontal pocketing.

Because of this well-known behavior of gingiva in health and after periodontal surgery, it is often desirable to obtain physiologic contours in the bone during surgery that parallel the anticipated post-surgical gingival form. Osseous resective surgery (osteoplasty and/or ostectomy) achieves this goal. The indications for definitive osseous resective surgery are limited, however, because the therapist may

BIOLOGIC WIDTH

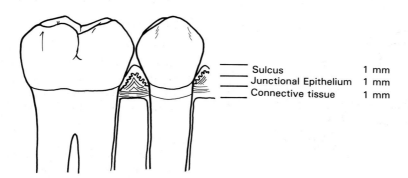

Sulcus   1 mm
Junctional Epithelium   1 mm
Connective tissue   1 mm

Fig. 16–8.

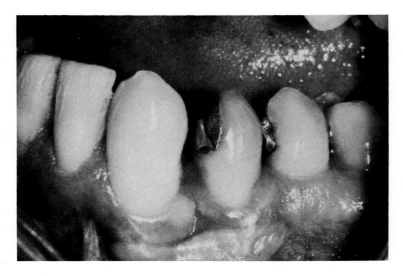

Fig. 16–9.

risk the removal of excessive tooth support and lessen the prognosis of the adjacent teeth.

Osseous Resection: Osteoplasty/Ostectomy

Osteoplasty is the removal of non-tooth-supporting bone to improve physiologic contour. Often large amounts of bone can be removed without the loss of tooth-supporting bone. Ostectomy is the removal of bone that is supporting the tooth (bone containing Sharpey's fibers of the periodontal ligament).

Indications

Osseous resective surgery has limited indications. The use of osteoplasty/ostectomy beyond these indications will sacrifice valuable tooth support, which is necessary for long-term tooth retention. Osseous resection is indicated in the presence of:

1. Shallow infrabony defects (1 to 2 mm in depth).
2. Class 1 and selected Class II furcation involvement.
3. Flat or reverse architecture, tori, exostoses, and ledges.

4. Bone contouring in conjunction with root resection.
5. Primary closure of flaps in conservative new attachment and replaced flap procedures.

Contraindications

There are times in periodontal surgery when osseous resection to achieve physiologic osseous contours results in the removal of too much bone and compromises the overall goals of therapy. The following are situations when osseous resection is contraindicated.

1. *Esthetics.* Removal of bone in maxillary anterior areas will result in an unacceptable esthetic result for most patients.
2. *Isolated deep defect.* Too much tooth-supporting bone would have to be removed from the adjacent teeth to obtain physiologic contours.
3. *Advanced periodontitis.* Teeth in these patients are already in a compromised situation. Additional removal of tooth-supporting bone would be contraindicated.
4. *Local anatomic factors.* Ascending ramus, external oblique ridge, max-

illary sinus, and flat palate are some of the anatomic factors that limit the chances of achieving physiologic osseous contours.

5. *High caries index.* Any procedure that results in additional exposure of root surfaces would not be indicated in these patients.

6. *Systemic conditions.* Health problems that limit osseous resective surgery would limit performance of all periodontal surgical procedures.

Technique

After adequate local anesthesia, a mucoperiosteal (full-thickness) flap is designed and performed as discussed in Chapter 14. The apically positioned flap is the technique most applicable when pocket elimination surgery and osseous resection is anticipated. Flap reflection should be adequate for visibility and access to the osseous defects. All granulomatous tissue should be removed by using sharp curets. All calculus should be removed from the tooth and the roots should be planed.

The first step in osseous resection is to thin the alveolar housing. The facial and lingual surfaces of the bone are reduced to provide a ramping effect into the interproximal areas where the osseous defects occurred, and to thin the bone over the facial and lingual surfaces of the teeth. This bone contouring is usually done with large round burs (Ns. 6 or 8) in a high-speed handpiece and cooled with sterile physiologic saline or sterile water. The second step in osseous resection is to flatten the interproximal defects by removing the coronal edges. This step is also usually done with rotary instruments. Please note that at this point, a reasonable amount of bone may have already been removed, but none of it was tooth supporting.

A situation has been established in which the interproximal bone is apical to the bone on the facial and lingual surfaces

of the teeth. In the third step, this facial and lingual bone is now removed with chisels to achieve a physiologic contour similar to that anticipated in the healed gingiva. A back-action chisel aids in removing bone at the distal line angles of the teeth.

The mucoperiosteal flap is then positioned and sutured to cover the bone and to contact the tooth about 1 mm coronal to the bone. An appropriate surgical dressing may be placed over the surgical site. Routine postoperative care for surgical patients is discussed in Chapter 11.

Effect of Bone Removal

Visual Effect

The bone is reduced to the depth of the interproximal defect. The supporting bone is removed primarily on facial and lingual surfaces; this usually amounts to an average of 0.6 mm of bone circumferentially and 1 to 2 mm of bone on the facial and lingual aspects. Because the facial surface is a highly visible area, the loss of bone appears to be magnified. Of course, where esthetics are a problem, osseous resection should not be done.

Effect on Tooth Mobility

Increased tooth mobility can be expected immediately after most periodontal surgical procedures. After adequate healing and tissue maturation, mobility will usually return to presurgical levels. A similar pattern follows osseous resection; after 6 to 12 months, mobility patterns also return to presurgical levels.

Lingual Approach to Osseous Resection

There are advantages to performing the bulk of the osseous removal from the lingual aspect in both the maxillary and mandibular arches. In the maxillary arch, the osseous defects can be ramped to the palate, which avoids removing bone from the vulnerable facial furcation areas. A wider area for access to perform the sur-

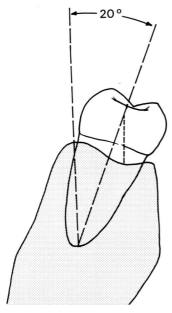

Fig. 16–10.

gery is thus maintained. The palatal approach also provides better access for oral hygiene postoperatively, and markedly improves the esthetic result.

In the mandibular arch, the teeth have a normal inclination lingually, which places the deepest point of most osseous defects in a lingual position (Fig. 16–10). Ramping the osseous defects to the lingual aspect requires less removal of tooth-supporting bone, which preserves the bone over an already coronally located facial furcation. The bone on the lingual surface, however, is often quite thick, and considerable effort is required to achieve the desired physiologic contours (Fig. 16–10).

Modified Osseous Resection

Due to the limitations associated with osseous resection, it is often impossible to achieve ideal physiologic contours in treating advanced periodontal disease. When defects are deep, many therapists modify the amount of bone removed to retain tooth-supporting bone in areas in which they believe it cannot be sacrificed. With this option, reversed or flat contours remain; an admitted compromise, but necessary to achieve maximal retention of functional teeth in a state of periodontal health that can be maintained.

Advantages of Osseous Resection

1. *Predictability.* By obtaining physiologic osseous contours at the time of surgery, the therapist knows the outcome of the procedure without having to rely on an unpredictable amount of bony fill and new attachment.
2. *Minimal waiting period.* After a reasonable healing period (8 to 12 weeks), gingival contours are at their best and restorative dentistry can be completed.
3. *Plaque control.* With the periodontal pocket eliminated or reduced to a minimum, the patient has access to root surface that previously had been within the periodontal pocket. The improved access enables the patient to clean the dentogingival areas adequately to maintain periodontal health.

Disadvantages of Osseous Resection

1. *Loss of attachment.* By design, the procedure removes bony attachment to achieve the desired result. The loss of attachment may be lessened by the use of a lingual approach or a modification of the technique.
2. *Esthetics.* Additional clinical crown length is less desirable than teeth with a normal gingival position. Resective techniques should not be used in areas in which esthetics is of prime consideration.

Future Considerations

Periodontics is changing rapidly. As the profession becomes successful in controlling the pathologic microflora and predictable regenerative treatment modalities are developed, resective surgery will decrease in importance. For today, however, osseous resection provides dentistry with a predictable method of reducing periodontal pockets to a level that may be easily maintained by the patient and the dental professional.

CHAPTER 17

Management of Osseous Defects: Grafting

For many years, researchers and clinicians alike have attempted to regenerate lost osseous architecture by promoting regeneration of bone with various osseous stimulators. Bovine bone, cartilage, plaster of paris, cementum, dentin, fresh and preserved allografts, freeze-dried bone allografts, and autografts have been tried with varied success. To date, autografts and some allografts offer the best hope for inducing restoration of lost bone and regeneration of a functional attachment apparatus of the periodontium on a predictable basis.

INDICATIONS FOR BONE GRAFTING

Patient Selection

Patient selection is of critical importance when resorting to regenerative graft procedures. The factors causing the inflammatory periodontal disease must be controlled before reparative procedures are attempted. The patient must demonstrate effective oral hygiene, have no compromising physical or mental conditions, have a positive attitude toward therapy, and be amenable to a long-term post-therapy maintenance program.

Defect Selection

The osseous morphology to be grafted is as important as patient selection. Realistic expectations of success are directly proportional to the number of osseous walls remaining in the defect, and is inversely related to the number of avascular tooth walls. A narrow (less than 2 mm wide), three-wall defect confined to a single tooth surface has great inherent osseous regenerative potential without resorting to bone grafts. A wide (more than 2 mm), three-wall defect confined to one or more surfaces of the tooth, a two-wall or one-wall defect, or combinations of the foregoing has progressively less inherent osseous potential, and bone grafting may regenerate some lost support. The least predictable situations for osseous regeneration are furcation defects and supracrestal regeneration of bone.

TYPES OF GRAFTS
Autografts

Autogenous bone grafts are of two general types: free osseous autografts and contiguous autografts.

Free Osseous Autografts

Free autografts may be composed of cortical, cancellous, or combined cortical-cancellous bone. Clinical experience suggests that the less dense composition of cancellous bone affords greater opportunity for success, but it is often more difficult to obtain and its supply may be meager. Consequently, the majority of defects are filled with a combination, cortical-cancellous bone, with the higher percentage usually being cortical bone. Autografts can be obtained from extraoral or intraoral sites.

Extraoral Donor Sites. Autogenous hemopoietic marrow/cancellous bone has been used in grafting of periodontal defects for over 15 years. It is obtained from the ilium by a cut-down procedure or by a punch biopsy technique from the anterior or posterior superior iliac crest. The cores of marrow and cancellous bone may be used fresh or may be stored for various periods. The iliac marrow/cancellous bone may be stored for up to 2 weeks when refrigerated at 4°C in minimum essential media. For longer periods, the autograft can be placed in a combination of minimum essential media and glycerol and frozen in a conventional freezer. When used after refrigeration or freezing, the material is rapidly warmed to body temperture before implantation.

The basic functions of all grafting materials are as follows.

1. Osteoconduction. The graft acts as a template or trellis to assist in bone formation.
2. Osteoinduction. The graft acts to stimulate or to induce new bone formation.
3. Osteogenesis. The cells of the graft actually produce new bone.

Studies have consistently shown that bone marrow grafts have extremely high osteogenic potential. Fresh hemopoietic marrow differs from other grafting materials in that it contains numerous pluripotential cells, which may differentiate, proliferate, and actually participate in bone formation. The extent to which they participate is unknown. It has been shown that refrigerated or frozen marrow, in which the stem cell vitality has been reduced, appears to be osteogenically equal to fresh marrow.

Bone marrow autografts have been used successfully in the treatment of one-, two-, or three-wall infrabony defects and some furcation involvement. Alveolar crestal heights have been increased in a few reported cases, and in several instances alveolar dehiscence has been repaired.

Bone marrow has shown great promise in periodontal therapy, but it does have some disadvantages. In most instances, the services of a physician are required to obtain the material, and the experience is time-consuming, costly, and often traumatic for the patient. The punch biopsy method for obtaining the marrow is less traumatic than the cut-down procedure, but some patients express considerable apprehension about submitting to either procedure. The major problem reported with fresh iliac marrow/cancellous bone is progressive root resorption. Some clinicians have noticed extensive tooth resorption coronal to the crestal area of the implant for as long a time as 1 year after successful bone fill. Resorption of this type is rarely observed with intraoral autogenous bone or when the hip marrow/cancellous bone is refrigerated or frozen for delayed transplantation. The reasons for this resorption are only speculative.

Intraoral Donor Sites. Bone that is removed during osteoplasty/ostectomy is an excellent source of material. The size of the chips may vary from fairly large fragments to small particles, depending on how the bone removal is performed. If rotary instruments are used, the particle size is small. There is evidence that the small particles of donor bone may more actively induce regeneration in osseous defects. Small particles offer the advantage over large fragments of a greater surface area for resorption and then replacement by new host bone.

A technique has been described in which a large, round carbide bur revolving at 25,000 to 30,000 rpm is used to reduce bone to small particle size during osteoplasty/ostectomy. This fine donor bone is gathered and, when mixed with the patient's blood, forms a coagulum, that is placed in the defect. A surprising amount of bone can be obtained from cortical bone shavings obtained when performing osteoplasty and ostectomy procedures or reducing the bulk of supporting bone or tori. Instruments especially useful are chisels (Ochsenbein, Wedelstaedt) or files (Chigo, Sugarman).

A method to reduce cortical and/or cancellous bone fragments to a smaller size and a plastic consistency by utilizing the mechanical amalgam triturator is called the bone blend technique. The large particle, intraoral donor bone is placed in a sterile unused plastic amalgam capsule with the pestle and is triturated for 30 to 60 seconds. This action reduces the larger particles to the consistency of slush, which can be easily placed and molded into an osseous defect.

Bone may be obtained from a healing socket 6 to 12 weeks after an extraction. A flap is made over the socket. The cancellous bone/marrow slush is then harvested from the socket with rongeurs or large curets and is placed in the osseous defect. The immature bone and cells appear to offer excellent healing and reparative potential.

Bone may also be obtained from maxillary tuberosities, edentulous ridges, or retromolar areas. Usually a window is made in the outer cortical bone for access to the cancellous areas. Cancellous bone from the tuberosities once contained hemopoietic marrow, but in the adult, this hemopoietic content is minimal. Limited visual and mechanical access, together with the frequent occurrence of an alveolar extension of the maxillary sinus in the tuberosity, severely reduces the availability of graft material in this region.

Contiguous Osseous Autografts

This type of autograft is seldom used to eliminate osseous defect (bone swaging). The technique involves the use of a green-stick fracture of bone compressing the bone into the defect.

Allografts

An allograft is a tissue graft between individuals of the same species. Use of allografts may give some inductive capacity comparable to autografts, but allografts may initiate graft rejection by the host. Examples of allografts include freeze-dried bone, frozen hemopoietic marrow/cancellous bone, and merthiolate-treated bone. The bone tissue should be procured under rigid conditions to ensure it is an aseptic donation of tissue that is free of any transmissible pathologic conditions.

Freeze-Dried Bone

Considerable research on the use of freeze-dried bone in periodontal osseous defects has been conducted by the U.S. Navy Tissue Bank over the past 10 to 15 years. After following rigid criteria for donor selection and processing, the freeze-dried bone is ground to 100 to 300 μm average particle size and is placed in sterile bottles with an indefinite shelf life. Considerable testing of this material has demonstrated the allograft to be nonantigenic. Some allograft materials are decalcified with the intent of increasing osteogenic potential. The advantage of using allografts over autografts is that there is no need to create an additional surgical wound to procure donor material and still maintain comparable osseous induction potential.

Alloplastic Grafts

Alloplastic grafts are synthetic substances, the most promising of which, for periodontal use, are ceramic materials. Currently available are porous, resorbable B-tricalcium phosphate (Syntho-graft) and dense, nonresorbable hydrox-yapatite (Calcitite, Periograft) grafts. Histologic research efforts suggest these substances are essentially biocompatible fillers, with little evidence of bone or attachment apparatus regeneration. Clinical results do suggest that these materials may effectively fill the defect and thus help maintain bone and soft tissue height. There are no biologic or clinical advantages to the use of alloplastic grafts in comparison with allografts or autografts.

Composite Grafts

Composite grafts are usually combinations of autogenous graft material and an allograft or alloplast. Because a form of autogenous bone is the preferred graft material, and at times the amount available is insufficient to meet the needs, expander in the form of an allograft or alloplast is used to extend the supply. There is some evidence to indicate that the composites form more new bone than either of the components of the composites grafted independently.

SURGICAL PROCEDURES

The technique for preparation of the recipient bed is the same regardless of what donor material is utilized.

1. Make an extracrevicular scalloped, internally beveled incision around the neck of the teeth to remove the sulcular epithelium and the inner soft tissue walls of the pocket. Preserve as much gingival tissue as possible to ensure primary closure of the wound.
2. Elevate a mucoperiosteal (full-thickness) or a mucosal (partial-thickness) flap to expose the defect. Occasionally, one or more relaxing incisions

may be needed to provide better access.
3. Remove all soft tissue fibers and granulomatous tissue from within and around the osseous defect.
4. Plane the root surface until smooth and hard.
5. Intramarrow penetrations with a sharp instrument or a No. ½ round bur may be performed. The compact bone that lines the defect is perforated to allow for rapid growth of new blood vessels into the area from the surrounding marrow. Intramarrow penetration also permits bone-forming cells to enter the graft site.
6. The graft material is firmly placed into the defect at or only slightly coronal to the existing osseous walls.
7. Replace the flaps over the graft and suture. Be sure to approximate the wound edges interproximally to ensure primary flap closure.
8. Place a suitable periodontal dressing over the surgical area.
9. Postoperative instruction should be given to the patient to minimize pain and swelling (see Chapter 11).
10. Remove sutures after 7 to 10 days, debride the wound, and polish the involved teeth. Redress if necessary.
11. After final dressing removal, instruct the patient in plaque control. Biweekly professional plaque debridement for several months after surgery enhances your final results. Do not probe the graft sites for at least 3 months.

Note: An antibiotic regimen is prescribed for the first 10 to 14 days of healing (tetracycline hydrochloride—250 mg every 6 hours). Studies have shown that results are enhanced if therapeutic levels of tetracycline are maintained for plaque suppression during the first week of healing.

CHAPTER 18

Management of Osseous Defects: Furcation Involvement

TREATMENT CONSIDERATIONS

Philosophy

Treatment of teeth with furcation involvement complicates periodontal treatment. A furcation involvement may be defined as a pathologic condition that has destroyed the periodontium in the intraradicular area of a multirooted tooth. Treatment of these teeth has varied from conservative maintenance to extraction. Recently, the trend has been toward retaining these teeth, especially if they are of strategic importance in the overall treatment plan. Nevertheless, the dentist is cautioned to avoid unnecessary heroics in attempting to salvage seriously involved, multirooted teeth by means of "interesting" techniques. Before attempting extensive therapy, the dentist should ask the following questions.

1. Can a morphologic environment be established that can be adequately maintained by the patient?
2. Will retention of this tooth preserve arch integrity and obviate prosthetic replacement?
3. Will retention permit better prosthetic design?
4. Is the tooth vital to an existing prosthesis?

5. Can the proposed therapeutic effort be considered realistic therapy?

Diagnosis

Pathologic conditions in this area are diagnosed by the use of a periodontal probe, a pigtail or cowhorn explorer, and radiography. The use of radiography must be related to the clinical examination. For example, radiographic examinations may reveal evidence of a furcation involvement, whereas probing reveals that the soft tissue attachment is still intact, with *no* entrance into the furcation area. Obviously, the clinical examination is the critical evaluation in this instance.

Maxillary molars with extensive pocket depth (5 mm or more) on the mesial, distal, or midfacial aspect should automatically be suspected of having furcation involvement. In mandibular molars, extensive midfacial or midlingual pocket formation strongly suggests an intraradicular pathologic process, regardless of the radiographic evidence.

Probing and positive identification of maxillary furcation involvement can be especially difficult. Occasionally, local anesthesia must be employed to permit adequate diagnosis. The mesial entry to the furca is best accomplished from the palatal aspect. The distal entry may be

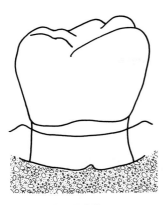

CLASS I

Fig. 18–1.

accomplished from either the palatal or the facial aspect. Although careful presurgical diagnosis can minimize the possibility of an unexpected, "surprise" furcation problem, final, positive evidence is often found only at the time of surgery.

Classification

Classification of furcation pathology can be divided into four grades: Grade I (incipient defects), Grade II (moderate involvement), Grade III, and Grade IV (through-and-through communication). These grades may be defined in greater detail.

Grade I. A soft tissue lesion extending to the furcation level but with minimal osseous destruction. Radiography of these incipient lesions reveals little, if any, evidence of a pathologic condition (Fig. 18–1).

Grade II. A soft tissue lesion combined with bone loss that permits a probe or explorer to enter the furcation from one aspect but not to pass completely through the furcation. This grade is further subdivided as follows.

Degree I. Greater than 1 mm and less than 3 mm of horizontal penetration of bone loss in the furcation.

Degree II. Horizontal loss of 3 mm or greater but no through-and-through involvement (Fig. 18–2).

Grade III. Lesion with extensive osseous destruction that permits through-and-through communication covered by soft tissue (Fig. 18–3).

Grade IV. The through-and-through furcation involvement is clinically exposed and open. There is complete visualization through the furcation (Fig. 18–4).

Prognosis

The prognosis of teeth with a furcation involvement depends on the following factors.

1. Extent of horizontal and vertical bone destruction in the intraradicular space.
2. Number of roots, their morphology, and furcal roof morphology.
3. Morphology of the intraradicular space (width, depth, etc.).
4. Health status of the periodontal ligament (determined by tooth mobility, percussive response, etc.).
5. Access for surgical correction.
6. Access for plaque control by the patient after surgical correction.
7. Pulpal status and prospects for successful endodontics therapy and root removal procedures.
8. Ability to control occlusal factors.
9. History of caries.

When the foregoing factors are equal, mandibular first molars generally have the best prognosis, followed by mandibular second molars and maxillary first molars. The prognosis of maxillary premolars is considered poor, even when there is only moderate furcation involvement. Anatomically, premolar teeth do not lend themselves to satisfactory plaque control or to root amputation. The possibility of new attachment in the furcation area, with or without osseous grafting, is not a highly predictable procedure.

Pulpal-Periodontal Relationships

The relationship between pulpal disease and periodontal disease has been in-

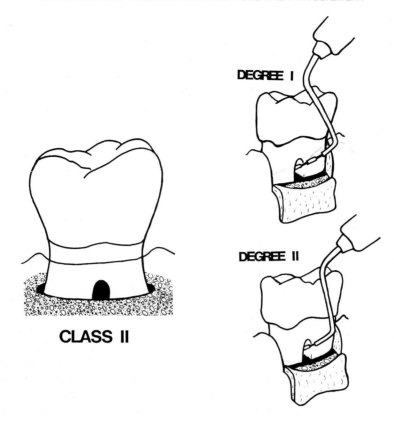

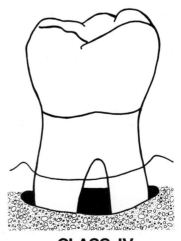

DEGREE I

DEGREE II

CLASS II

Fig. 18—2.

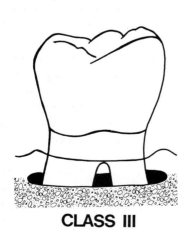

CLASS III

Fig. 18—3.

CLASS IV

Fig. 18—4.

creasingly appreciated. It is apparent that there are many direct communications between pulpal tissue and the periodontal ligament. Dentists cannot consider these areas as separate and unrelated environments. Therefore, in diagnostic terms, a pulpal evaluation should be a part of every periodontal examination.

Pulpal-periodontal interaction is especially important in intraradicular areas. Because of the potential accessor foramina in the furcation areas, Grade II and Grade III furcation lesions are sometimes associated with pulpal disease. It has been demonstrated that the intraradicular periodontal apparatus is especially sensitive to excessive occlusal stress. Thus, the combination of pulpal disease, periodontal traumatism, and inflammatory periodontitis might reasonably be expected to produce extensive destruction in the furcation area.

The potential for pulpal-periodontal interrelationships provides continual diagnostic challenges to the therapist. The clinician must be highly suspicious of pulpal disease, especially when the following conditions exist:

1. Periodontal pockets near or leading to the furcation area or apex.
2. Sinus tract of uncertain origin.
3. Discolored teeth.
4. Chronic drainage from the sulcus.
5. History of acute or chronic pulpal insult (periodontal traumatism, extensive restorative dentistry, etc.).
6. Prolonged hypersensitivity.
7. Evidence of slow or inadequate healing of periodontal lesions.

THERAPY

Grade I Involvement

Treatment for incipient furcation lesions is essentially the same as for an uncomplicated soft tissue pocket. *If* the width of attached gingiva is adequate (see Chapters 1 and 15), gingivectomy/gingivoplasty/odontoplasty may be employed, together with thorough debridement and root preparation. The surgery is accomplished to permit access to the furcation for both the therapist and patient.

1. Careful attention should be given to the character of the cervical crown area. Inadequate Class IV restorations, cervical caries, and poor crown contours may be predisposing factors that should be corrected.
2. Projections of enamel into the furcation area may influence the spread of gingival inflammation. This anomaly occurs on the buccal aspect of about 25% of all molars. Although the importance of such projections is not clear, the therapist should be aware of them. Removal of the enamel projections by odontoplasty may be indicated, especially if new attachment is anticipated. On the other hand, if the furcation is left permanently exposed, removal of these anomalies may cause unnecessary tooth sensitivity.

Grade II Involvement

The prognosis and treatment approach are related to the severity of the Grade II furcation involvement.

Degree I. The prognosis for maintaining a furcation with this severity of involvement is good. Therapy will vary from conservative root preparation to surgical access of the furcal area for osseous surgery. Furcation plasty may be necessary for maintenance of oral hygiene by the patient.

Degree II. The prognosis for maintaining a furca with this severity of involvement is less favorable than a Degree I involved tooth. In addition to the procedures for the Degree I furcation, a more aggressive approach (root resection or hemidissection) may be required.

Grades III and IV

There are several categories of therapy for Grade III and Grade IV furcation involvement. These involve:

1. Increasing the furcation opening to facilitate plaque control.
2. Eliminating the furcation by various root removal procedures.
3. Extracting the tooth.

Attempts to reestablish total furcation integrity—bone, periodontal attachment apparatus, and dentogingival relationship—by bone grafting continue to represent an unpredictable form of treatment.

Furcation Plasty

Enlargement of an existing Class III furcation defect may facilitate plaque control and permit retention of the tooth. Enlargement may be at the expense of the tooth structure, the bone, or both. This approach, however, is generally limited to mandibular molars. Occasionally, a trifurcation area can be opened widely, but adequate plaque removal is difficult. Even after successful treatment of the Class III furcation involvement, caries in the furcation area is a constant threat. Caries control is essential for success in the treatment of *all* furcation involvement. The use of the various topical fluorides is recommended.

Root Resection

Root amputation is a predictable procedure for Class III trifurcation involvement. The root with the greatest overall bone loss is the logical candidate for amputation. If there is no marked difference, the D-B root is most likely for removal. The M-B root is most desirable for retention because of favorable root size and position in alveolar bone (Fig. 18–5). There are several points to consider before root resection.

1. The therapist should study root and furcation anatomy on extracted molars.

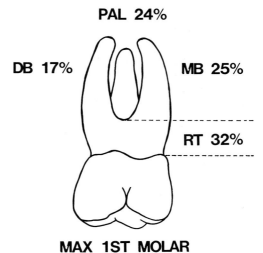

PAL 24%

DB 17%   **MB 25%**

RT 32%

MAX 1ST MOLAR

Fig. 18–5.

2. Occlusion should be checked and adjusted. The occlusal table should be narrowed, and/or lateral occlusal forces should be removed (Fig. 18–6).
3. The need for splinting should be established.
4. The strategic importance of teeth indicated for root resection should be thoroughly evaluated.

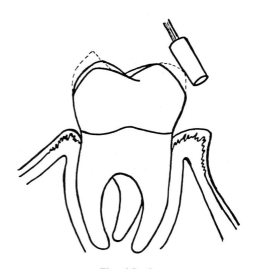

Fig. 18–6.

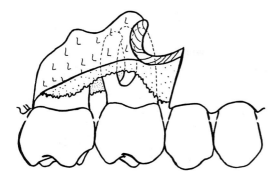

Fig. 18–7.

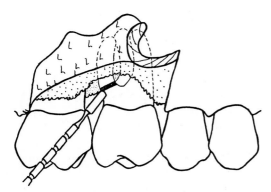

Fig. 18–8.

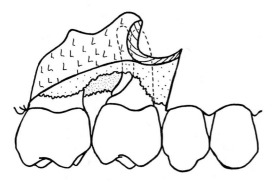

Fig. 18–9.

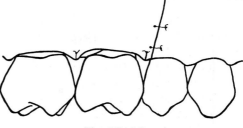

Fig. 18–10.

5. The maxillary sinus should be located and avoided.

Technique

1. Elevate a full-thickness flap to expose the defect (Fig. 18–7). Relaxing incisions may be required for adequate access and tissue placement.
2. Make the initial cut on the root with an appropriate bur apical to the cementoenamel junction, beginning in the furcation area. Amputation should be at the expense of the root rather than of the crown (Fig. 18–8).
3. Remove the root.
4. Contour the resected root stump. The root surface must be tapered to permit complete access by the patient (Fig. 18–9).
5. Suture the flap (Fig. 18–10) and cover with a periodontal dressing.
6. Remove suture in 1 week and recheck contour.
7. Polish stump with a fluoride-containing polishing agent.
8. Accomplish endodontic therapy before or soon after (within 2 weeks) root amputation.

Hemisection

Hemisection involves the removal of one half of the tooth. The same technique is used as was described for root resection. The retained root can often serve as a suitable abutment for fixed splinting.

CHAPTER 19

Management of Osseous Defects: Additional Techniques and Summary

SCALING, ROOT PLANING, AND PLAQUE CONTROL

Ideally, deep periodontal pockets and osseous defects should be reduced to permit patients to accomplish effective plaque control and to arrest the disease process. If this is not possible, for whatever reason, management by scaling, root planing, and plaque control should be considered. It is unlikely that such pockets are ever successfully "managed" by scaling and root planing. It is more likely that the frequent removal of subgingival plaque and calculus simply retards the rate of progression of periodontal disease. If this therapy is to be of any value, scaling and root planing must be accomplished at frequent intervals (every 2 to 3 months); in the interim, the patient must accomplish meticulous plaque control. The advantages of retaining teeth with deep pockets must be carefully weighed against the possible disadvantages, such as potential abscess formation or loss of adjacent bone from sound teeth.

Indications

Some of the more common conditions in which scaling and root planing alone can be utilized are:

1. A patient who does not or cannot accomplish effective plaque control, but for whom extractions are not presently indicated.
2. A medically compromised patient.
3. A patient with periodontal disease who will not agree to periodontal surgery or extraction.
4. A strategic but severely involved tooth that is functioning as an abutment for a fixed or removable partial denture.
5. Extensive generalized bone loss in an elderly patient.
6. A patient with extreme fear of periodontal surgery.
7. Extensive bone loss around a single tooth in an intact arch, where retention does not jeopardize adjacent teeth.

SELECTIVE EXTRACTION

There are those clinicians who believe the only predictable method of treating periodontal disease is extraction of the involved teeth. This philosophy can be likened to that of the physician who believes the only predictable treatment for a hangnail is amputation of the finger, because hangnails are prone to recur. Extraction represents the ultimate failure in dentistry; yet, on occasion it can be used to advantage.

Selective extraction (strategic extraction) of some periodontally involved teeth can significantly improve the prognosis of adjacent teeth. For example, in Figure 19–1, severe periodontal involvement of this vital right first premolar has also resulted in bone loss of the adjacent teeth. The tooth exhibits Class III mobility and its prognosis is poor. If it is extracted, the socket will fill approximately to the highest level of the alveolar crest on the adjacent teeth, as shown in Figure 19–1. Consequently, the extraction of one tooth with a poor prognosis results in an improved prognosis for the adjacent teeth. Selective extraction is a consistent and predictable method of case management. It is a technique to be *used, but not abused* (Fig. 19–1).

FLAP CURETTAGE/DEBRIDEMENT

Several reports have suggested that thorough surgical debridement of osseous defects and adjacent pathologic root surfaces may result in some bony fill

of the defects. Replaced full-thickness flaps coupled with defect debridement for osseous regeneration appear to work best in narrow three-wall defects. Critical to maximizing the bony repair is thorough and frequent professional and personal plaque control after surgery.

MINOR TOOTH MOVEMENT

Orthodontic tooth movement can create favorable alterations of gingival form and osseous morphology. These changes often modify the extent of or even eliminate the need for pocket reduction surgery. Teeth can be moved into a vertical bony defect to narrow the lesion and improve the chances for success with regenerative techniques. Teeth can also be moved away from the osseous defect (such as in molar-uprighting techniques), thereby leveling the bone and modifying or eliminating the bony defects. Similarly, forced eruption can be used to modify the osseous topography. Some corrective osseous surgery is frequently needed after the forced eruption to finalize the hard tissue and soft tissue contours. Further

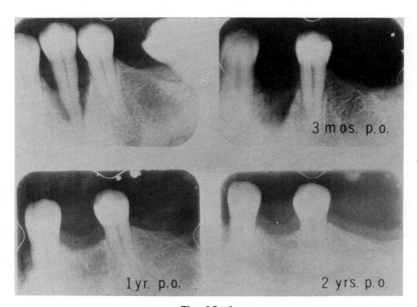

3 mos. p.o.

1 yr. p.o.

2 yrs. p.o.

Fig. 19–1.

details related to the integration of orthodontics and periodontics are provided in Chapter 8.

ROOT SUBMERGENCE

Recent research and clinical reports have suggested that submergence of either vital or root canal-treated roots may result in regeneration of bone and subsequent maintenance of the alveolar ridge. The periodontal surgical technique is similar to bone grafting or flap curettage techniques, emphasizing thorough root detoxification and defect debridement. The teeth are severed at or apical to the alveolar crest. The flaps are sutured to achieve primary wound closure and coverage of the root stumps.

SUMMARY OF TREATMENT OF OSSEOUS DEFECTS

The prognosis of infrabony pockets is influenced by the number of remaining osseous walls, the size of the defect, the number of root surfaces involved, the extent of bony destruction, and the furcation involvement. As a general rule, the greater the number of osseous walls and the narrower the defect, the better the prognosis for new attachment will be, provided there is no furcation involvement. A summary of therapy for various osseous defects follows.

1. Broad interproximal ledges (lipping)—osteoplasty.
2. Abrupt interproximal irregularities of bone—osteoplasty.
3. Exostoses that interfere with pocket elimination or proper flap closure—osteoplasty.
4. Three-wall defect
   a. Narrow
      (1) Bone grafts
      (2) Flap curettage
   b. Broad (wide-mouthed): bone graft
5. Two-wall defect

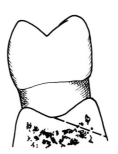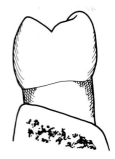

Fig. 19–2.

   a. Shallow crater
      (1) Osteoplasty/ostectomy (Fig.19–2)
      (2) Flap curettage
   b. Deep crater
      (1) Bone graft
      (2) Flap curettage
      (3) Combined procedures including osteoplasty-ostectomy, defect debridement, and/or bone grafts
6. One-wall defect
   a. Shallow—osteoplasty/ostectomy, if adjacent tooth is not jeopardized. Otherwise, use bone graft technique.
   b. Deep
      (1) Bone grafts
      (2) Combined procedures
7. Combination defect—Combination procedures
8. Grade I furcation involvement
   a. Scaling and root planing
   b. Gingivectomy/gingivoplasty
   c. Osteoplasty/ostectomy plus odontoplasty
9. Grade II furcation involvement
   a. Osteoplasty/ostectomy and odontoplasty
   b. Root resection/hemisection
   c. Bone grafts
10. Grade III furcation involvement
    a. Root resection/hemisection
    b. Osteoplasty/ostectomy with odontoplasty to open defect through and through for plaque control.

CHAPTER 20

Periodontal Emergencies

A periodontal emergency is any circumstance, or a combination of circumstances, that adversely affects the periodontium and requires immediate attention. This definition encompasses a wide variety of conditions that involve the periodontium; however, this discussion will be limited to the emergencies most often encountered.

PERICORONITIS

Etiology

Pericoronitis is probably the most common periodontal emergency, and the partially erupted or impacted mandibular third molar is the site most frequently involved. The overlying gingival flap is an excellent harbor for the accumulation of debris and an ideal breeding ground for bacteria. Additional insult to the pericoronal flap is often produced by trauma from an opposing tooth.

Signs and Symptoms

The clinical picture is a red, swollen, possibly suppurating lesion that is extremely painful to the touch. Swelling of the cheek at the angle of the jaw, early necrotizing ulcerative gingivitis, partial trismus, lymphadenopathy, and radiating pains to the ear are common findings. The patient may also have systemic complications such as fever, leukocytosis, and general malaise.

Treatment

The treatment of pericoronitis consists of irrigation of the undersurface of the flap and the surrounding area with warm saline solution. A 10-ml syringe with a *blunt* 10-gauge needle, bent at an 80° angle, is an excellent irrigating instrument. An ultrasonic instrument can also be used effectively in this region. It may be necessary to extract the opposing third molar at the first visit if it impinges on the pericoronal flap. The patient is instructed to rinse with warm salt water every 2 hours, and antibiotics are administered if systemic complications are present. Once the acute symptoms have subsided, a careful evaluation is made to determine whether the tooth should be retained and whether further periodontal therapy is indicated to alter the environment.

ABSCESS FORMATION

Gingival Abscess

A gingival abscess is a localized (usually superficial), painful, rapidly expanding lesion that appears suddenly in the marginal gingiva or interdental papilla. The lesion consists of a purulent focus in connective tissue. It is initiated by the forceful embedding into the gingiva or gingival sulcus of a foreign body (e.g., a toothbrush bristle or popcorn husk). A gingival abscess may occur in tissue entirely free from periodontal disease.

Treatment consists of drainage to relieve the acute symptoms and removal of the foreign body. If the lesion has become fluctuant, topical anesthesia is applied to the gingival margin. The gingival sulcus is gently opened with a curet to permit evacuation of pus, the sulcus is gently instrumented, and copious amounts of warm saline are used to flush the area. The patient is advised to rinse with warm salt water every 2 hours. Once the irritant is removed and drainage is established, the tissues usually return to normal with no further treatment.

Periodontal Abscess

A periodontal abscess is a localized, purulent inflammatory process involving the deeper periodontal structures. Abscess formation is usually associated with infrabony pockets, deep tortuous pockets, and furcation involvement. Conditions that either force material into deep pockets, prevent free drainage, or occlude the orifice of a pocket may result in abscess formation. The latter may occur when patients become conscientious about plaque control and improve the tissue health in the marginal area without treatment of the deeper problem.

Periodontal abscesses may be acute or chronic. Acute lesions often subside and persist in the chronic state, while chronic lesions may suddenly become acute. The clinical signs of an acute abscess are severe pain, swelling of the soft tissues, tenderness to percussion, extrusion, and mobility of the involved tooth. Periodontal destruction in an acute abscess may be rapid and extensive, and treatment should be instituted promptly.

Treatment of the periodontal abscess is performed in two stages. The first stage involves management of the acute symptoms by drainage. Whenever possible, drainage is established through the lumen of the pocket. If this cannot be done, as is often the case when there is a furcation involvement or a tortuous pocket, drainage is obtained externally by making a stab wound through the pointed lesion. The patient is advised to rinse with warm salt water every 2 hours and antibiotics are prescribed if systemic complications are present. It may often be necessary to adjust the occlusion of the involved tooth or teeth.

The second phase of treatment is directed toward elimination of the pocket as soon as the acute symptoms have subsided and before the chronic stage is reached. Treatment consists of careful elevation of a mucoperiosteal flap. All granulomatous tissue is removed and the root surface is lightly planed. Emphasis is placed on gentle manipulation of the soft tissue. The flap is replaced in its original position and sutured. A periodontal dressing is used for 7 to 10 days. Clinical experience has demonstrated a marked propensity for healing and repair after acute periodontal destruction. For this reason, teeth affected by an acute periodontal abscess should be carefully evaluated before extraction is recommended.

Acute Periapical Abscess

It is sometimes necessary to differentiate between a periodontal and periapical abscess. A nonvital pulp is usually indicative of a periapical abscess, and the tooth should be either treated endodontically or extracted. A clinically responsive vital pulp is not always assurance that the problem is still not pulpal. Radiography is of some assistance in differential diagnosis, but clinical findings such as extensive caries, tooth vitality testing, pocket formation, and continuity between the abscess and the gingival margin are of greater practical significance.

Various investigators have confirmed pulpal pathosis and infection in periodontally involved teeth. Thus, the probability exists that periodontitis can result in death of the pulp. It has also been demonstrated that, as a result of pulpal disease, tissue destruction may proceed from the apical region toward the gingival margin. This process is termed retrograde periodontitis to differentiate it from marginal periodontitis, in which the disease spreads from the gingival margin to the apex. Whether the periodontal pocket is a result of retrograde or marginal periodontitis, or a combination of both, is academic. In all cases, treatment should consist of either combined endodontic-periodontal therapy or extraction of the tooth.

CHEMICAL AND PHYSICAL INJURIES

Injuries caused by toothbrush trauma, chemical burns, cheek and tongue biting, factitious habits, and periodontal dressings are occasionally observed. Emergencies of this type are painful but otherwise of little consequence. Healing usually occurs uneventfully in 10 days to 2 weeks. Treatment is chiefly symptomatic, and patient discomfort is controlled through the use of topical anesthetics or warm saline rinses.

NECROTIZING ULCERATIVE GINGIVITIS

History

Necrotizing ulcerative gingivitis (NUG) is an emergency of special importance. As long ago as 400 B.C., Greek soldiers were plagued by what appears to have been NUG. In the 1890s, Plaut and Vincent were the first to associate specific organisms with the disease process, hence, the term Vincent's infection has been associated with the disease for many years. The condition is also called Vincent's stomatitis, Plaut-Vincent's disease, Plaut-Vincent's stomatitis, trench mouth, and many other names. Because the trend in dental

and medical terminology is to dispense with the use of eponyms, the descriptive term "necrotizing ulcerative gingivitis" is preferred.

Incidence

An increase in NUG among college students after final examinations and periods of stress has been reported. NUG has also been related to cigarette smoking, increased consumption of alcohol, low socioeconomic status, poor nutrition, age, general debilitation, and climate. In effect, any factor that increases emotional stress, lowers patient resistance, or inhibits plaque control can contribute to the initiation of NUG.

Contagion

For many years, NUG was considered to be a communicable disease contracted from eating utensils, personal contact, etc. Numerous studies have failed to establish any pattern of transmission among individuals. Some hardy investigators have even injected fusospirochetal microorganisms in their own mouths and have not contracted the disease. The 1966 World Workshop in Periodontics concluded, on the basis of existing evidence, that NUG was not a communicable disease.

Etiology

The etiology of NUG can be divided into predisposing and causative factors.

1. *Predisposing factors.* Local factors include calculus, gingival flaps over molar teeth, caries, overhanging margins of restorations, improper tooth contacts, malpositioned teeth, and food impaction. Systemic predisposing factors include emotional stress, heavy alcohol intake, cigarette smoking, fatigue, malnutrition, and general debilitation.
2. *Causative factors.* These are microorganisms. The acute disease develops from a host-parasite imbalance as a result of an overwhelming in-

crease in the number of bacteria and/or lowered patient resistance. Organisms that have been associated with NUG are *Bacillus fusiformis, Borrelia vincentii,* α-hemolytic streptococci, *Bacteroides melaninogenicus,* and other unidentified vibrios, spirochetes, and streptococci. It is interesting to note that the number of spirochetes is proportional to the amount of inflammation and the amount of necrosis present. Current research has shown organisms penetrating the tissue in the lesions of NUG. Even though a specific organism has not been conclusively demonstrated to produce NUG, it has been well established that microorganims are the exciting causative agents of the disease. The dramatic response to antibiotics, both topical and systemic, is valid evidence of the role of bacteria in the etiology of NUG. Once antibiotic administration is stopped, the disease usually recurs unless the predisposing factors have been eliminated.

Diagnosis

NUG can be diagnosed on the basis of clinical findings alone. The onset of the disease is manifested quite suddenly, and patients complain of severe pain about the teeth or gums. Usually, they cannot determine any one particular area that hurts but say, "My entire mouth hurts," or "All of my teeth hurt." The pain is more intense at the sites of ulceration. The second most prominent symptom experienced by the patient is bleeding gums. Bleeding is often spontaneous, and patients may observe blood on their pillows or notice the taste of blood when they awaken. Patients may also experience marked pain and bleeding while brushing their teeth or when eating. Alcoholic beverages, hot or cold liquids, or spicy foods may be intolerable.

The most characteristic and pathog-nomonic finding of NUG is ulceration and cratering of the interdental papillae (Fig. 20–1). Frequently, the papillae are reduced to punched-out masses of necrotic tissue covered by a gray-white pseudomembrane. Acute pain and bleeding result from the slightest pressure on the area. Ulcerated areas spread by contiguity and by contact. The mucosa of the lips, the jaws, and the palate may be affected, and ulcerated areas may be found on the tongue. The fetid odor of necrosis is usually present, but this distinctive odor is not pathognomonic of NUG in that it may be present in any site of tissue necrosis. There may or may not be a number of systemic findings. Fever, headache, general malaise, loss of appetite, and regional lymphadenopathy may be present. The constitutional symptoms seem to parallel the severity of the disease and are usually more pronounced in younger individuals.

Differential Diagnosis

A number of diseases produce lesions similar to those of NUG. Lesions most commonly mistaken for NUG include those of acute gingivitis, primary herpetic gingivostomatitis, recurrent aphthous stomatitis, desquamative gingivitis, infectious mononucleosis, acute leukemia, agranulocytosis, and the secondary stage of syphilis. Only NUG, however, produces ulceration and cratering of the interdental papillae. It should be emphasized that NUG can occur in conjunction with any number of systemic debilitating diseases.

1. *Acute gingivitis* (Fig. 20–2). An intense generalized or even localized acute gingivitis can mimic any of the signs and symptoms of NUG. In gingivitis, pain is not as severe nor as persistent, and rarely is there spontaneous bleeding. In many patients with acute gingivitis, the interproximal areas and gingival margins are filled with food, plaque, and materia alba. Once this debris is removed

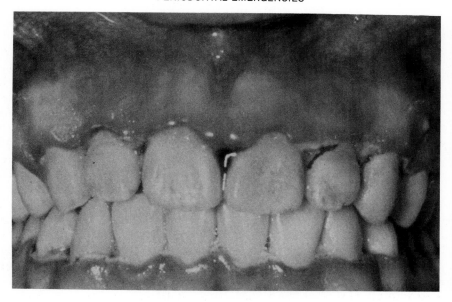

Fig. 20–1.

and the interproximal areas can be examined, the lack of necrosis and crater formation will verify the diagnosis of nonulcerative gingivitis.

2. *Primary acute herpetic gingivostomatitis* (Fig. 20–3). This disease is characterized by small ulcers with elevated, halo-like margins. The lesions are yellowish and cheesy in appearance and bleed less readily on pressure than does NUG. The lips, tongue, buccal mucosa, palate, gingiva, pharynx, and tonsils may be involved. The disease is accom-

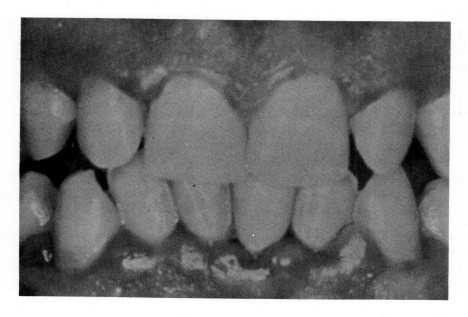

Fig. 20–2.

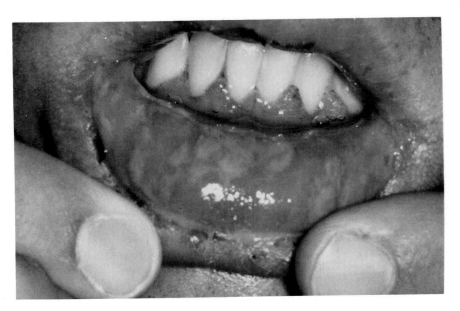

Fig. 20–3.

panied by generalized soreness, which interferes with eating or drinking. The typical interdental crater of NUG is lacking. Patients usually display rather severe systemic symptoms with typical herpetic lesions, extraorally and intraorally. Diagnosis is based on clinical findings and patient history. Acute herpetic gingivostomatitis usually runs a course of 7 to 10 days. Treatment consists of palliative measures. The patient is placed on a regimen of warm water rinses, soft diet, and forced fluids. Plaque and superficial calculus are removed to reduce gingival inflammation. If the patient experiences pain when eating, a 0.05% solution of dyclonine hydrochloride or viscous xylocaine may be prescribed for use before meals. It is swished in the mouth for about 2 minutes and then expectorated. Local anesthesia is produced and lasts up to 1 hour. Dyclonine hydrochloride can be used several times daily without fear of toxicity.

3. *Recurrent aphthous stomatitis*

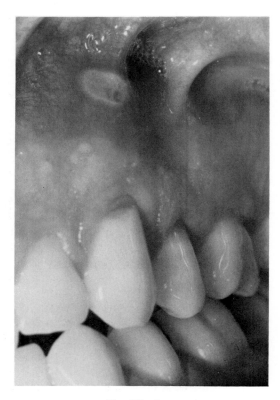

Fig. 20–4.

(canker sores) (Fig. 20–4). This condition is characterized by single or multiple epithelial erosions, which can occur on the buccal mucosa, lateral margin of the tongue, floor of the mouth, soft palate, and pharynx. The ulcers are covered by a gray-white membrane with an erythematous margin and minimal adjacent erythema. The condition is extremely painful, and one or more oral lesions may be present. Common precipitating factors include mucosal trauma, psychic stress, and endocrine imbalance. In patients who suffer continuously with this condition, a recommended treatment is tetracycline hydrochloride, oral suspension. One teaspoon containing 250 mg is swished around the mouth for 2 minutes and then swallowed. This is done four times daily for 5 days as soon as the prodromal signs are recognized. This treatment is not recommended for those individuals who experience only the occasional aphthae or who are sensitive to tetracyclines.

4. Chronic desquamative gingivitis. This gingival condition is probably a clinical syndrome rather than a disease entity. The etiology is not known; however, the condition is probably an oral manifestation of a bullous dermatologic disease, such as benign mucous membrane pemphigoid or lichen planus. Desquamative gingivitis is most commonly observed in females (40 to 55 years old) and can occur in mild, moderate, and severe forms. In the mildest form, there is diffuse, painless erythema of the gingiva. In the moderate to severe form, there are scattered red and gray areas involving the marginal and attached gingiva. The gingiva can usually be rubbed off with finger massage or blown off with an air syringe (Nikolsky's sign), leaving a bleeding surface. The papillae do not undergo necrosis; therefore, there is no interdental cratering. The patients complain of a burning sensation, thermal sensitivity, and pain when brushing the teeth. The mild form of this condition may be painless, but the severe form is extremely painful. Diagnosis is based on clinical findings and biopsy. Local treatment consists of gentle prophylaxis, plaque control, and elimination of all forms of local irritants. In the most severe cases, topical and/or systemic corticosteroids are used to supplement the local therapy. Topical hormones are often effective supplements to local therapy: for female patients, a cream containing 1.25 mg/g of conjugated estrogen, and for males, methyltestosterone ointment, 2 mg/g. Some therapists have successfully eliminated the condition by gingivectomy.

5. Infectious mononucleosis. This benign infectious disease is usually seen in children and young adults. The symptoms include a sudden onset of fever, nausea, headache, vomiting, malaise, loss of appetite, swelling, and tenderness of the lymph nodes. The patient often complains first of a sore mouth and throat. Orally, there may be diffuse erythema of the mucosa and petechiae. The marginal gingiva and interdental papillae are swollen, inflamed, and bleed spontaneously or upon gentle pressure. There is no ulceration or interdental crater formation, but secondary development of NUG affords a diagnostic challenge. Diagnosis is based on hematologic and immunologic findings.

6. Leukemia (Fig. 20–5). Oral manifestations occur with great frequency in patients with leukemia, particularly acute and subacute monocytic leukemia. Clinical changes may vary

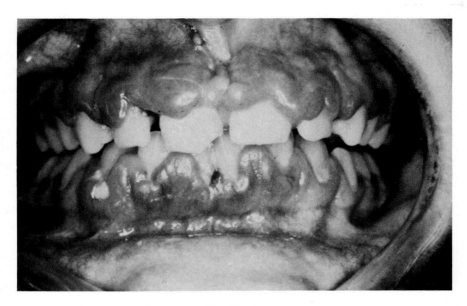

Fig. 20–5.

from a diffuse cyanotic discoloration of the entire gingival mucosa to a tumorous gingival enlargement. The enlargement may be localized or generalized, diffuse or marginal; but in all cases it is associated with local irritants, such as plaque, calculus, faulty restorations, and trauma. The clinical signs of NUG are often superimposed upon leukemic gingival enlargement. When there is a lack of response to local treatment of NUG, a complete blood count, urinalysis, and bone marrow studies are essential to rule out the presence of leukemia and other blood dyscrasias.

7. *Agranulocytosis (malignant neutropenia).* This condition is manifested orally as ulceration and necrosis of the gingiva, which resembles NUG. The ulcers are covered by a gray or gray-black membrane, but there is less inflammation associated with the lesions of agranulocytosis than NUG. Lesions are also observed in the oral mucosa, tonsils, and pharynx. The most common cause is a reaction to a wide variety of drugs. Diagnosis is based on blood studies and bone marrow biopsy.

8. *Secondary syphilis (mucous patch).* The oral lesions of syphilis are usually on the tongue, the gingiva, or the buccal mucosa. They are usually ovoid or irregularly shaped and are surrounded by an erythematous zone. The mucous patch rarely affects the marginal gingiva, and the overlying gray-white plaque is not detachable. The lesions are usually painless but are highly infectious. Diagnosis is made by positive results of serologic analysis and dark-field examination of an affected lymph node.

Treatment

The dentist should attempt to: 1) control the acute bacterial phase; 2) educate the patient in plaque control; and 3) eliminate the predisposing factors, both local and systemic. Early and vigorous local treatment during the acute phase will produce rapid and dramatic results in most cases. Drugs should never be considered a substitute for scaling and debridement. Antibiotics should be used only when systemic complications are evidenced.

Basic steps in treatment are as follows:
First Visit
1. Remove as much calculus, plaque, and debris as possible, as soon as possible, and as gently as possible. Ultrasonic instrumentation is the method of choice because it provides irrigation and debridement.
2. Instruct the patient in plaque control. Begin patient education and motivation. Have the patient hold their soft brush under warm water to soften the bristles further and then instruct in the use of the brush.
3. Antibiotics may be administered systemically if there is evidence of elevated temperature, lymphadenopathy, and general malaise. Most cases do not require antibiotics. Mild analgesics may be prescribed for pain.
4. Instruct the patient in home care. It is advisable to give the patient a mimeographed sheet of specific instructions for other procedures to be followed at home.

Recommended Home Care Instructions for the Patient
1. Rinse the mouth vigorously with warm saline solution (1 level teaspoon of table salt dissolved in 1 glass [8 oz.] of warm water) every 2 hours.
2. Follow a soft, bland diet of milk, eggnog, broth, etc. Dietary supplements (Nutrament, Metrecal, Carnation Instant Breakfasts, etc.) are especially useful during this period.
3. Drink plenty of water.
4. Avoid foods that are hard, fried, coarse, spicy, or starchy.
5. Reduce or eliminate smoking and drinking of alcoholic beverages.
6. Rest as much as possible.
7. After eating, rinse the mouth with warm saline solution.
8. Brush the teeth in the manner prescribed.
9. Return to the dental office after 24 hours.

Second Visit
1. Check oral hygiene and review plaque control procedures.
2. Continue removal of calculus, plaque, and debris.
3. Polish the teeth.
4. Have patient return after 24 to 48 hours.

Third Visit
1. Check plaque control. Review procedures, if indicated.
2. Continue elimination of all irritants, which includes all calculus, overhanging margins, open contacts, etc.
3. If the tissues have not responded dramatically by the third visit (48 to 72 hours), evaluate for systemic factors (leukemia, infectious mononucleosis, etc.). Refer for medical consultation, if necessary.
4. If improvement is apparent, make an appointment for reevaluation in 1 week; otherwise continue to see the patient every 24 to 48 hours.

Fourth Visit
1. Check plaque control.
2. Check for calculus and debris.
3. Evaluate for further periodontal therapy.

NUG responds rapidly and dramatically to local therapy and effective plaque control. As a result, some patients and clinicians become somewhat complacent about the severity of the disease. It is important to remember, and to caution the patient accordingly, that unless the treatment is continued to completion, NUG is likely to recur. Likewise, uncontrolled NUG can result in localized osteonecrosis, extensive soft tissue destruction, or even Ludwig's angina has been observed in cases of infectious mononucleosis, acute leukemia, and uncontrolled diabetes. For this reason, if there has not been a dramatic response to the local treatment of NUG by 72 hours, the patient should be referred for medical consultation.

HYPERSENSITIVITY

Hypersensitivity is often a management problem for both the patient and the dentist. This is true despite the wide variety of medicaments and desensitizing paraphernalia available.

Etiology

Hypersensitivity of exposed dentin can occur when dentinal tubules are exposed either by caries, fracture, periodontal disease, or periodontal instrumentation. Trauma from occlusion is also a frequent cause of hypersensitivity. Under such circumstances, thermal stimuli (hot or cold foods), chemical stimuli (sweet or sour foods), and tactile stimuli (toothbrushes and dental instruments) can excite a painful response. It is most discouraging to the patient—and futile for the dentist—to insist upon vigorous plaque control when the procedures are painful.

Treatment

Hypersensitivity can be controlled by eliminating the etiologic factors and by using desensitizing agents. There are several patient-applied and dentist-applied preparations, all of which have some degree of success. One of the first treatments to be considered, especially after surgical procedures, should be occlusal adjustment. Even a slightly heavy occlusal contact can make a tooth or teeth in a recently treated area very sensitive. Refinement of the occlusal contacts often renders immediate relief.

Patient-applied commercial products can be very effective. Strontium chloride- and potassium nitrate-containing toothpastes may be used as medicaments, applied for 1 to 1½ minutes after regular plaque-control procedures. Relief should be achieved within 1 week.

Dentist-applied medicaments include ophthalmic suspensions of prednisolone acetate, sodium fluoride solution, and dibasic calcium phosphate. Each of these are applied after the sensitive area is polished with flour of pumice. The medicament is then applied with a cotton pledget or porte polisher. Several applications may be needed to achieve complete relief. Local anesthesia may be required before applying the medicaments. Refractory cases may require root canal therapy if the tooth is to be retained.

PRIMARY PERIODONTAL TRAUMATISM

Definition

Primary periodontal traumatism is the condition in which tissue injury (trauma from occlusion) is produced in an otherwise normal periodontium by excessive occlusal force (traumatogenic occlusion). Secondary periodontal traumatism is the condition in which relatively normal occlusal forces produce injury in a weakened periodontium. Microscopically, both conditions may appear the same. The periodontal ligament demonstrates necrosis, hemorrhage, thrombosis of blood vessels, and dissolution of principal fibers and there is bone loss and widening of the periodontal ligament space. It should be reemphasized that excessive occlusal stress does not initiate gingivitis and pocket formation.

Signs and Symptoms

Traumatogenic occlusion may result in pain on chewing, tenderness to percussion, and sensitivity to temperature change. The traumatized tooth is often mobile. In such instances, the pain is localized and is usually associated with the recent insertion of a restoration or a dental appliance, with parafunctional habits, or with a recent injury to the jaw or teeth.

If the tooth is vital, it is frequently hypersensitive to electrical stimuli.

If excessive occlusal forces are of long duration, the tooth or teeth are mobile, but usually there is little or no pain when chewing and little response to percussion. Migration of the traumatized tooth is frequently observed. The patient complains of increasing thermal sensitivity and occasionally a dull, aching sensation. Diagnosis can often be made by placing the index finger over the mobile tooth and having the patient glide into working and nonworking excursions. The tooth will move in and out of alignment as the excursions are accomplished (fremitus).

Treatment

Treatment of primary periodontal traumatism consists of eliminating the etiologic factor or factors; this may entail selective grinding of the teeth or removal of the irritating appliance. When the cause was a severe blow, it may be necessary to splint the teeth until the acute symptoms have subsided. Bite guards have been used effectively to manage this problem. Once the traumatogenic force is eliminated, the potential for complete reversibility of the lesion is good. In most cases, root sensitivity will disappear after adjustment of the occlusion. Desensitizing solution is often applied to afford immediate relief of the sensitivity and to encourage plaque control.

TEMPOROMANDIBULAR JOINT (TMJ) PAIN DYSFUNCTION SYNDROME

Etiology

Injury to the TMJ and the muscles related to the function of the joint may result from an extrinsic source, such as a traumatic blow, or from an intrinsic source, such as a muscle spasm. It is not within the scope of this chapter to discuss the multitude of signs, symptoms, etiologic factors, and therapies proposed for TMJ dysfunctions; however, it is important that all dentists have a basic understanding of this extremely painful and demoralizing condition. It is generally, but not universally, agreed that the cause of the dysfunction pain is a combination of psychic tension and occlusal disharmony. These factors together result in hyperactivity and pain in the masticatory muscles and dysfunction of the jaw. There is no evidence to show organic changes of the joint, except for degenerative arthritis; consequently, the sequelae are similar to those that occur in any joint complex after longstanding functional disorder.

Symptoms

The clinical syndrome is associated with five symptoms, which may vary from patient to patient:

1. Pain in the region of the TMJ, ear, face, and neck.
2. Cracking or popping noises associated with TMJ movement.
3. Limitation or deviation of mandibular movement (muscle spasm).
4. Subluxation or dislocation of the mandible.
5. Difficulty in mastication of food.

Treatment

Many forms of therapy have been proposed for this problem, and some success has been reported with most methods. Studies continue to indicate that psychologic factors play a major role in the onset of most TMJ problems. Consequently, many clinicians are adopting techniques that do not result in irreversible alterations of teeth, muscle, or joint structures, yet afford successful treatment. The following approach is recommended as one concerted but effective method of management of TMJ pain dysfunction syndrome.

1. Talk and listen to the patient. Diagnose the problem. Always take a positive approach to patient man-

agement. Assure the patient that the problem can be corrected.

2. Make an impression for a bite guard as soon as possible.

3. When there is extensive trismus, prescribe a tranquilizer until the trismus subsides. Diazepam (5-mg tablets) is specific for this problem and is the drug of choice, if one is needed. It is administered by asking the patient to take one tablet in the morning and one tablet in the evening.

4. Instruct the patient to:
   a. Limit mandibular movements.
   b. Eat a soft diet; avoid incising foods; chew bilaterally.
   c. Avoid yawning. This can be accomplished by clasping the hands on the back of the neck and pulling forward with the arms when the urge to yawn arises. This forces inspiration and will usually prevent yawning.
   d. Apply warm, moist heat as often as possible (four to six times daily).
   e. Avoid teeth clenching, pipe smoking, fingernail biting, etc.
   f. Relax by walking, jogging, playing tennis, and taking hot showers, hot baths, and sauna baths.
   g. Sleep on your back.

5. Insert and adjust the bite guard as quickly as possible.

6. Tell the patient to wear the bite guard 24 hours daily, removing it only to accomplish plaque control.

7. Once the acute symptoms have subsided, ask the patient to continue to wear the bite guard during sleep and during periods of stress.

CHAPTER 21

Periodontal Consideration in Restorative Dentistry

All phases of restorative dentistry are dependent on the establishment and maintenance of periodontal health to ensure lasting benefit. In this chapter, the term restorative dentistry encompasses the restoration of individual teeth to normal contour and function. Considerations relating to operative dentistry and fixed and removable prosthodontics are included.

TOOTH PREPARATION

Operative dentistry should be performed as atraumatically as possible to avoid permanent damage to the periodontium. The completed restoration should not interfere with plaque control, should not promote food impaction, and should be compatible with the patient's optimal occlusion. The restoration should be easily cleaned by the patient, a feature that requires well-fitting margins and a smooth finish.

NARROW BAND OF ATTACHED GINGIVA

The health and functional potential of the gingiva should be considered when the margin of a crown or Class V restoration is to be placed subgingivally. If the zone of attached gingiva is inadequate or minimal, the gingival margin is likely to recede after tooth preparation, gingival retraction, impression making, and placement of temporary restorations. These problems can be avoided by placing restoration margins coronal to the gingival margin (Fig. 21–1), but the requirements for retention and the location of caries frequently preclude this approach. Another solution would be to create surgically a wider band of attached gingiva at the site before restoration. As mentioned in Chapter 15, this gain in attached gingiva can be established with free soft tissue grafts or laterally positioned flaps.

WEDGES

Care should be taken not to lacerate the gingival tissues when placing matrix bands or wedges. Carelessly placed wedges may cause unintentional papillectomy. Use of a rubber dam helps prevent such damage, but the rubber dam clamps also can be destructive if improperly positioned on tissue rather than teeth.

RETRACTION STRINGS

Impregnated strings used for gingival retraction can injure the gingiva if left in

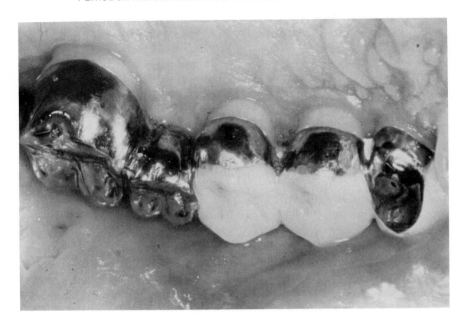

Fig. 21–1.

place too long or if the gingival tissues are inflamed before retraction. The effects of the chemicals in the retraction strings cannot be controlled. *Pressure retraction of the gingiva with chemical-free strings is recommended whenever possible.* The vasoconstrictor (8% racemic epinephrine) in some impregnated retraction string is rapidly absorbed and can cause a transient elevation of blood pressure and blood sugar. Vasoconstrictor-impregnated strings are contraindicated in patients with coronary disease, diabetes, hyperthyroidism, or severe hypertension. The maximal dose of epinephrine for a healthy patient is 0.2 mg, but epinephrine-containing strings contain 0.5 to 1.0 mg per inch (2.54 cm). Again, it is highly recommended that cords that do not depend on adrenergic drugs be substituted for retraction purposes.

CONTOURS

Tooth contours should be such that food is shed away from the gingival mar-

gins during mastication. Teeth are naturally shaped to prevent food from contacting the gingival margins during the masticatory occlusal stroke. Overcontouring encourages stagnation of food in the gingival sulcus and will interfere with plaque control procedures. Restoration of normal tooth contour should be a major objective of the restorative dentist (Fig. 21–2).

MARGINAL RIDGE

Approximating marginal ridges should be even in height, and well-defined occlusal fossae should be developed in the restoration. Such refinements help prevent the wedging of food interproximally. An inconsistent relationship of the marginal ridges is the factor most frequently associated with food impaction. When the maxillary anterior teeth are restored with full coverage, lingual cingula should be developed to shunt incised food away from the palatal gingival margin.

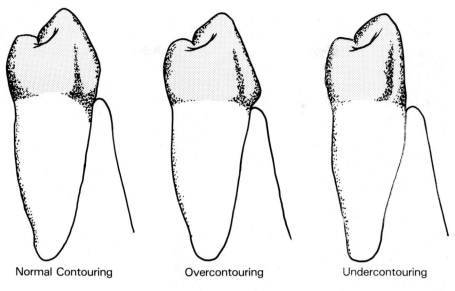

Normal Contouring   Overcontouring   Undercontouring

Fig. 21–2.

EMBRASURES

The gingival embrasure is usually occupied by the interdental papillae in patients who have never experienced periodontal disease. During the progress of plaque-related periodontal disease or after periodontal treatment, bone and soft tissue are lost and the interdental space is opened. It is advisable to place restorations that preserve the morphology of the crown and root and maintain the enlarged embrasure. The height, width, and faciolingual depth of the embrasure must be maintained. The proximal surfaces of restorations should:

1. Taper away from the contact area. Broad contact areas crowd out the interdental papillae and reduce access for plaque control. The papillae become prominent and entrap food debris; crowding of the papillae leads to plaque related inflammation.

2. Be slightly convex. Concave contours make plaque control difficult.

3. Extend the contact faciolingually to

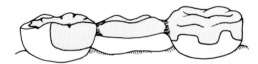

Fig. 21–3.

a degree that prevents food impaction.

4. Be as smooth as possible.

FIXED PARTIAL DENTURES

When missing teeth are replaced by fixed partial dentures, the abutment teeth must carry an increased burden, which can further compromise abutments already weakened by periodontal disease. This burden may be eased somewhat by 1) directing occlusal forces primarily along the long axes of the teeth, and 2) including a sufficient number of teeth in the prosthesis to distribute occlusal forces over as many abutments as possible.

Fixed partial dentures complicate plaque control by the patient. When esthetics permit, the use of a sanitary

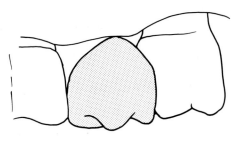

Fig. 21–4.

hygienic pontic (Fig. 21–3) or a bullet-shaped spheroidal pontic (Fig. 21–4) provides better access for plaque control. In the anterior region, the modified ridge lap pontic (Fig. 21–5) meets esthetic demands and yet can be readily cleansed. The patient may require auxiliary devices, such as bridge cleaners, twisted wire "needles," interproximal brushes (which are particularly effective when space permits), or floss threaders. It is the responsibility of the dental team to teach patients the proper use of these devices.

Fixed partial dentures should be designed so that every surface can be readily cleansed; this necessitates the inclusion of convex surfaces and open embrasures. The position of solder joints can be critical; they should be located as far away from the gingiva as possible to permit proper embrasure form. These joints should not be bulky.

Overhanging margins lead to damage of the periodontium. The damage occurs because they provide breeding sites for microorganisms that are inaccessible to

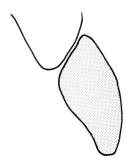

Fig. 21–5.

the patient's plaque-control devices. An overhanging margin should be recontoured and smoothed, or the restoration should be replaced.

Care must be taken to remove all excess cement from the gingival sulcus and/or pontic. Retained cement particles act as an irritant and can result in plaque retention, inflammation, and pocket formation.

REMOVABLE PARTIAL DENTURES

The design of removable partial dentures should enhance masticatory efficiency and esthetics without damaging the remaining teeth and supporting structures. Particular care is needed in the design of distal extension, removable partial dentures. In these appliances, abutment teeth are expected to receive—and survive—heavy, multidirectional forces. Such concepts as the altered-cast technique, the mesio-occlusal rest, the I-bar clasp, the guiding plane, and meticulous adjustment of the framework are all based on consideration for the remaining teeth.

Regardless of the restorations placed, all patients should be instructed and motivated to control bacterial plaque. Those individuals who receive fixed or removable partial dentures should be given specific instructions concerning plaque-control problems they will encounter. Patients must be instructed to remove plaque routinely from all surfaces of a removable appliance as diligently as they cleanse their teeth. Frequent evaluation is necessary to ensure patient effectiveness and cooperation.

CROWN-LENGTHENING PROCEDURES

The surgical lengthening of the clinical crown is required in certain situations. These include: subgingival caries, short clinical crown, clinical crown fracture, revision of an existing crown preparation, crown preparation requiring deep subgingival amalgam, and subgingival perforation. In general, these clinical situations may result in the margins of a fixed restoration intruding into the important "biologic width" zone of the root surface. This zone includes the space coronal to the alveolar crest for: the sulcus (1 to 2 mm); the junctional epithelium (1 mm); and the connective tissue attachment (1 mm). Unless allowance is made for this critical width in a preparation close to the alveolar bone, a poor gingival response and/or further bone loss will result. During the periodontal surgical procedure, a dimension of about 3.5 to 4 mm should be created between the proposed new restoration margin and the alveolar crest.

The apically positioned flap, with osseous resection, is the procedure usually used for crown lengthening. After surgery, about 8 to 10 weeks should be allowed for healing and maturation of the attachment apparatus (including re-formation of the gingival sulcus) before final tooth preparation and impressions are performed.

CHAPTER 22

The Role of Occlusion in Periodontal Health and Disease

The stomatognathic (gnathostomatic) system consists of the temporomandibular joints, neuromusculature of the masticatory apparatus, and the teeth within the periodontium. This chapter addresses the role that occlusion plays on the periodontium.

The primary causes of periodontitis are micro-organic (bacterial plaque and their by-products); the role that occlusion plays in the initiation and progression of the disease process is secondary. Trauma from occlusion may alter or modify the progress of periodontal disease, but does not initiate the inflammatory lesion.

First, it is important that a few terms be defined.

1. *Trauma from Occlusion (occlusal trauma).* The injury produced in the periodontium by occlusal forces exceeding the adaptive capacity of the periodontium. The injury may manifest clinically by mobility, migration of the teeth away from the force, and pain during biting or percussion. Radiographically, the injury may be identified by a discontinuity of the lamina dura at the lateral aspects and around the apices of the involved teeth. A widening of the periodontal ligament space may or may not be evident.

2. *Primary Occlusal Trauma (Fig. 22–1).* An injury from an excessive occlusal force acting on a periodontium that has not been altered by disease (a healthy periodontium). Primary occlusal trauma is usually a result of excessive occlusal forces associated with such factors as parafunctional habits, high restorations, and removable partial dentures. There is no attachment loss. The lesion is reversible and can usually be corrected by eliminating the local factors (i.e., bacteria and their by-products) and/or by adjusting the occlusion.

3. *Secondary Occlusal Trauma (Fig. 22–2).* An injury from a normal occlusal force placed on a weakened periodontium. This is often observed after treatment of advanced cases of chronic destructive periodontitis. The greater the loss of periodontal support, the more important the occlusal factors become in the prognosis and treatment of the disease.

4. *Combined Periodontal Trauma.* An injury from an excessive occlusal force on a diseased periodontium. In effect, inflammation is present, pocket formation is present, and ex-

Primary Occlusal Traumatism

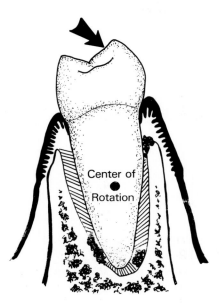

Fig. 22–1.

Secondary Occlusal Traumatism

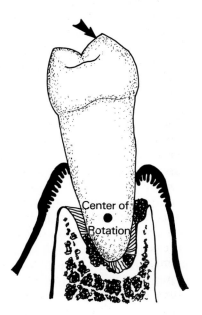

Fig. 22–2.

cessive occlusal forces exaggerate and/or exacerbate the disease process. Trauma from occlusion may be a co-destructive factor in combination with the existing active periodontal lesion. The resultant lesion is not reversible by occlusal adjustment.

Current research data provide overwhelming evidence that occlusal trauma will not cause periodontal pockets, and is not capable of initiating marginal gingival inflammation. Trauma from occlusion will not affect the progression of gingivitis to periodontitis. When there is an existing periodontitis and occlusal trauma is superimposed upon the active lesion, clinical and research evidence leads us to believe that these excessive occlusal forces do not allow the periodontium to adapt. Consequently, there may be an increase in the rate of spread of the inflammatory process into the underlying tissues. Trauma from occlusion, superimposed upon the active periodontal lesion, may result in deeper pockets and can contribute to angular bony defects.

There is some controversy regarding the concept that trauma from occlusion may contribute to the formation of angular defects. The role that trauma plays in the etiology of periodontal disease, according to one theory, is better understood if the periodontium is considered as two zones: the zone of irritation and the zone of co-destruction. The former consists of the soft tissue coronal to the alveolar crest fibers and transseptal fibers; the latter consists of the periodontium apical to the alveolar crest fibers and transseptal fibers (Fig. 22–3).

The inflammatory lesion (gingivitis and periodontitis) starts in the zone of irritation; this is caused primarily by irritation from bacteria and their toxic products. Trauma from occlusion does *not* cause gingivitis or periodontal pockets. The marginal gingiva is not affected by trauma from occlusion and as long as the

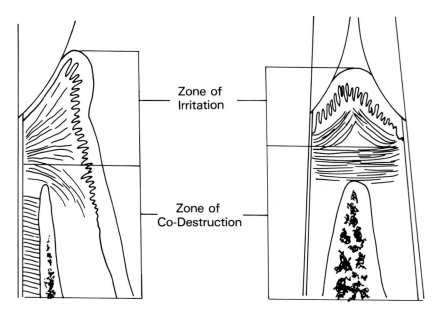

Fig. 22–3.

disease process is limited to the gingiva (zone of irritation), occlusal forces will not play a role in the pathogenesis of inflammatory periodontal disease.

When the inflammatory process extends into the alveolar process (into the zone of co-destruction), trauma from occlusion may play a role in the pathogenesis of the disease process. If the occlusal forces are unfavorable (excessive), this trauma may alter the environment and pathway of inflammation. These unfavorable forces may produce periodontal injury and thus become a co-destructive factor that may affect the pattern and severity of tissue destruction. There is a large amount of evidence to indicate that increased loss of alveolar bone and altered osseous morphology occur when trauma from occlusion is superimposed upon periodontitis.

In summary: 1) trauma from occlusion in the absence of gingival inflammation does *not* cause a pocket; 2) trauma from occlusion does not affect the loss of connective tissue attachment; 3) teeth move in the direction of the occlusal force; 4)

unilateral trauma may cause bone resorption on the pressure side and bone apposition on the tension side; and 5) bone loss may occur on all sides of a tooth or may be extensive enough to cause tooth mobility.

There are various approaches to treating trauma from occlusion. The most common methods are: 1) occlusal adjustment (equilibration), 2) bite plates (night guards, bite guards), 3) orthodontic tooth movement, 4) splints, and 5) reconstructive restorative dentistry. The primary goal of occlusal treatment is to establish harmony within the stomatognathic system. The overall primary goal of periodontal therapy, however, is to control the inflammatory response.

Occlusal adjustment is the technique most often used when minor occlusal therapy is indicated. The goals of occlusal adjustment are: 1) to remove occlusal prematurities in maximal intercuspation and centric relation, 2) to eliminate balancing side interferences that act as torquing forces and prevent freedom of lateral movements of the mandible, 3) to adjust working-side contacts to protect teeth with a weakened periodontium, and 4) to eliminate protrusive interferences.

Bite plates are most often used when patients present with signs of stomatognathic system breakdown caused by parafunctional habits (bruxism, clenching, etc.). Splinting may be necessary for patients who exhibit discomfort as a result of tooth mobility or hypermobility that interferes with masticatory function or increased mobility after periodontal therapy. Orthodontic treatment of the periodontal patient may be indicated to achieve a more acceptable occlusal relationship.

In most instances, it is desirable to perform occlusal therapy during the initial preparation phase (inflammatory control phase), but after root detoxification and the control of periodontal inflammation. If extensive fixed prosthodontic dentistry is to be used as an occlusal corrective measure, these procedures should be postponed to at least 30 to 60 days after periodontal surgery has been completed.

CHAPTER 23

Problems and Failures in Periodontal Therapy

It is appropriate in this syllabus to consider the prospects for long-term success or failure in the management of periodontal disease. Until recently, many dentists have misunderstood periodontal diagnosis and therapy and, unfortunately, have considered the likelihood of failure with their patients to be as great as that of success. This viewpoint is not justified today, when scientifically based periodontal therapy is at its most rational, predictable, and successful level. Nevertheless, the widespread persistence of the myth of "inevitability" of periodontal failure—leading inexorably to the edentulous state—is a major impediment to the performance of periodontal treatment by many general dental practitioners. Numerous surveys have shown that these general dentists devote only about 3 to 5% of their practice time to periodontal concerns. A number of controlled longitudinal studies of treated and untreated periodontal diseases have profoundly influenced current concepts of periodontal management. Specifically, these findings have had a direct, positive bearing on our perceptions of success and failure in relation to periodontal therapy.

Briefly, the long-term studies have shown that:

1. Treated and well-maintained periodontal cases have significantly less pocket depth, bone loss, and tooth mortality than diagnosed but untreated cases, or treated but poorly maintained cases.
2. Pocket elimination surgery and reattachment procedures reduce pockets equally.
3. The effects of a regular every 3-month professional maintenance program are more significant than differences between surgical procedures in determining long-term periodontal health.
4. Thorough root preparation and long-term periodic maintenance are the most important components of all periodontal treatment programs.

GENERAL CAUSES OF FAILURE

Most periodontal therapeutic failures are far from mysterious. Because most periodontitis is caused by local factors, unsatisfactory therapy generally can be attributed directly to failure to identify and eliminate those local factors. In everyday practice, relatively few cases have their origins in bizarre systemic derangements.

Of course, failure may be total or partial, reversible or irreversible. Areas that do not respond satisfactorily to initial treatment methods, for instance, probably should not be classified as failures. Frequently, even surgical corrections must be planned as multistage procedures to achieve pocket reduction and optimal tissue architecture.

Effective periodontal therapy implies comprehensive long-term patient management. Unlike carious lesions, which usually require placement of a single restoration, periodontal problems rarely respond to one-step treatment. What appears to be a success when evaluated after a few weeks may prove to be a total failure on scrutiny after 1 year.

The following are the most common causes of failure in periodontal case management. Most of these factors have been discussed in other chapters, but are reemphasized here to underscore their relationship to failure.

1. Failure to Establish an Effective Long-Term Maintenance Program

One of the major reasons for failure of periodontal therapy is the lack of an effective recall system. Periodontal patients *must* be reevaluated at least every 3 months. This sequence permits a careful examination of the tissues and an opportunity to determine the effectiveness of the patient's plaque control. If there is an indication of tissue breakdown and/or laxity in plaque control, reinforcement of basic principles will usually reverse the disease process. The reader is referred to Chapter 24 for a more extensive discussion of maintenance therapy.

2. Failure to Instruct Patient Adequately in Plaque Control

Failure to instruct a patient adequately in plaque control is considered by periodontists to be a principal reason for failure. This problem may have several roots:

a. The practitioner may be overconfident of his knowledge of advanced plaque-control philosophy, techniques, and effectiveness.

b. The practitioner may fail to communicate with and/or to motivate the patient effectively; fail to reinforce previous instructions; or fail to evaluate the adequacy of previous instructions.

c. The dentist may fail to utilize disclosing media for plaque visualization.

d. The dentist may fail to give adequate demonstrations of the use of the toothbrush, floss, and other plaque-control devices.

e. The crux of the problem may be the failure of the dentist, to believe—and thus failure to communicate—that the *patient's* personal plaque control efforts are just as vital to periodontal therapy as the *practitioner's* procedures. A dentist who does not practice rigid personal daily plaque control will not succeed in motivating patients to become effective "co-therapists" in treating their own disease.

The patient may lack the motivation, the dexterity, or the mentality to accomplish effective plaque control. Under these conditions, periodontal therapy will predictably fail. It is incumbent on the dentist and hygienist to note these problems and to develop innovative approaches to disease control.

3. Failure to Formulate and Operate from a Simple, Comprehensive Written Treatment Plan

Failure to allow sufficient time in the treatment plan to reevaluate the adequacy of current therapy unquestionably accounts for many treatment failures. The results of initial preparation must be carefully reevaluated to determine the necessity for surgery. Postoperative reevaluation is also necessary to determine the results of definitive treatment.

4. Failure to Survey and Eliminate Common Local Factors

The failure to survey and eliminate common local factors is universally regarded as a prime cause of failure in the therapy. The following local factors are significant in plaque accumulation and food impaction:

a. Calculus.
b. Open contacts (verify visually and with floss).
c. Rough restorations and overhanging margins.
d. Uneven, sharp, or nonexistent marginal ridges.
e. Plunger cusps (can induce wedging of opposing teeth and produce food impaction).
f. Overcontoured crowns, poorly designed pontics, and poorly designed removable partial dentures. In general, it can be stated that sooner or later, anything less than absolutely fastidious execution of restorative procedures can compromise the health of the periodontium.

5. Failures Related to Diagnostic Deficiencies

a. Failure to obtain an adequate health history and failure to discern possible systemic influences on periodontitis or on patient management can have disappointing or even disastrous consequences. The patient's general health status can change suddenly. Medications must be monitored constantly, and records must be updated.
b. Dentists frequently fail to use a calibrated probe to evaluate and then fail to *record* the depth and location of pockets. Ironically, they may be meticulous in their use of an explorer to search for caries.
c. Failure to use a special furcation probe in furcations may leave areas of serious involvement undetected.
d. Failure to obtain adequate radio-graphs or to interpret radiographs adequately are serious omissions in the evaluation and treatment of periodontal problems.
e. Failure to note such anatomic characteristics as abnormal frenum influence, width of attached gingiva, or root prominences with associated dehiscence and fenestration deformities may have unfortunate consequences after surgery.
f. Failure to identify and correct traumatogenic occlusal relationships, including centric pathway prematurities, nonworking side contact, parafunctional habits, plunger cusps, etc., will compromise therapy. Routine examination of occlusion on every patient is necessary.
g. Many total periodontal failures can be associated with failure to recognize and remove hopelessly involved teeth early in the treatment.
h. Failure to consider the influences of periapical or pulpal disease on periodontal therapy can result in unexpected complications or unexpected loss of strategic teeth. The intimate pulpal-periodontal relationship has been increasingly appreciated in recent years. Routine pulpal assessment is an important part of the periodontal diagnostic process.

6. Failures in Approach to Periodontal Surgery

The benefits of periodontal surgery are well documented. Properly planned and executed, these procedures can facilitate root detoxification and plaque control by reducing pockets and by improving contours and other anatomic relationships. When casually conceived, however, surgery can result in the most frustrating of failures.

a. Selection of inappropriate surgical techniques at the outset can only lead to unacceptable results.

b. Excision of all attached gingiva, leaving margins of alveolar mucosa, results in an unstable functional arrangement. If such a situation is anticipated, a flap procedure rather than a gingivectomy is indicated.

7. Failures in Surgical Technique

a. Inadequate debridement of deposits, granulomatous tissue, amalgam particles, and diseased cementum can cause delayed healing or surgical failure.

b. Ragged, torn tissue on flap edges resulting from careless design, dull or improper instruments, and generally poor technique can result in delayed healing and undesirable contours.

c. Failure to use an aseptic technique can result in postoperative infection and surgical failure.

d. Failure to approximate wound edges adequately to ensure healing by primary intention may result in failure of new attachment procedures and of osseous grafting techniques.

e. Failure to stabilize grafts and flaps leads to displacement, undesirable contours, or involution, and to unnecessary sequestration of bone— and pain.

f. Failure to use pressure coaptation of flaps and grafts after suturing may lead to formation of a large fibrin clot, resulting in downgrowth of the epithelial attachment and bulbous contours.

g. Inadvertently forcing the periodontal dressing beneath the flap may result in permanent tissue defects.

SUMMARY

An analysis of failures in periodontal therapy reveals a many-factored problem. Most failures, whether partial or complete, can be attributed to inadequacies of plaque control, diagnosis, surgical techniques, root preparation, or maintenance. The greatest single cause for periodontal treatment failure results from failure of the therapist to educate and motivate the patient to practice effective plaque control.

Above all, the successful, periodontally oriented practitioner must design a personalized, long-term periodontal maintenance program for each patient. The recall system is simply the *administrative* component of that maintenance plan. Intervals of 90 days must be considered the optimal level of frequency for the vast majority of post-surgical periodontal patients, on the basis of current research. Obviously some patients must be seen for professional plaque removal more frequently.

CHAPTER 24

Periodontal Maintenance Therapy

Scientific evidence clearly shows that periodontal treatment can be successful in the vast majority of patients. One of the major elements of successful periodontal treatment is an effective periodontal maintenance program.

RATIONALE FOR A PERIODONTAL MAINTENANCE PROGRAM

During the 1970s, a number of studies from the University of Michigan and the University of Gothenburg in Sweden were performed to evaluate the effectiveness of a variety of surgical techniques. Interestingly, no major differences were found between the surgical techniques, but the deciding factor between success or failure was in the frequency and thoroughness of the maintenance therapy provided by the practitioner. Patients who were recalled every 2 weeks to every 3 months and received professional prophylaxis, scaling, and oral hygiene reinforcement could be stabilized in periodontal health.

RECALL INTERVAL

The interval between recall appointments must be tailored to each patient's needs. Some of the recall sequences used are as follows:

A. *One-week interval*
1. Immediate post-surgical evaluation, to minimize the effects of plaque in wound healing.
2. Initial preparation (Phase I) for periodontal disease control.
3. Acute conditions.
   This interval is most appropriate in the acute therapy phase.
B. *Two-week interval*
1. Used to minimize the disease process in patients with inadequate oral hygiene.
2. May not be practical for an extended period because of the cost and the time involved.
C. *Three-month interval*
1. The most common recall after active periodontal therapy.
2. Depending on the patient's level of oral hygiene and disease activity, the interval can be either increased or decreased.

ELEMENTS OF A PERIODONTAL MAINTENANCE PROGRAM

Time

Maintenance is a demanding procedure, which if done thoroughly and properly (which is what the patient has the right to expect), takes time. Although it is not possible to project how long it will take in a specific situation, some well-managed and respected periodontal practices assign 60 minutes for the average maintenance appointment. The time involved, however, must be adjusted to the personal needs of the patient.

A significant amount of time may be spent during each appointment showing courtesy to and interest in the patient. This time is necessary and well spent; personal attention increases patient rapport and will help to build and maintain a practice. Figure 24–1 is an example of a form that provides an excellent method of recording data collected at the maintenance visit. The form also allows recording of treatment rendered and future recommendations.

History

Before treating or re-treating any patient, review of the medical history is mandatory. Patients may have serious changes in their medical status between appointments. Some of these medical problems can be life-threatening to the patient when under the stress of a routine dental appointment. It is also advisable to review the nature of the dental treatment the patient has previously received as well as the prognosis assigned to the dentition and individual teeth.

Examination

Before any therapy is performed, the current dental and periodontal status of the patient must be determined. An examination sequence should be followed that permits a thorough evaluation of the patient. The following sequence is one that has proven reliable for many practitioners.

1. *Tissue examination.* This is done before any plaque indicator (red or colored dye) is applied to the teeth and gingiva. Tissue color, contour, and consistency is observed. Record only those observations that vary from normal limits.

2. *Probing depths.* All areas are probed and the depths over 3 mm are recorded on the dental chart.

3. *Bleeding and/or suppuration sites.* After probing a small segment of the mouth, look for bleeding (and suppuration) sites. It is recommended that these be recorded by circling the probing depth in red. If bleeding occurs at a site with an unrecorded depth, simply circle the space where a recording would have been. Even shallow crevices can be infected and show bleeding upon probing. Identification and treatment of these areas ensures maintenance of periodontal health. By comparing bleeding sites from visit to visit, fluctuating problems can be observed, especially persistent and serious problem areas. Bleeding is a sign of existing disease and must be addressed in therapy. Areas that continually bleed are major problems demanding active treatment. Sites that bleed only occasionally also need immediate treatment, but they are not as significant a problem.

4. *Mobility.* Tooth movement is measured by applying force buccolingually between two dental instrument handles. Mobility should be recorded according to the criteria in Chapter 5.

5. *Furcations.* Health status of each furca should be determined and recorded.

6. *Caries.* At all recall appointments, examine for caries. Any or all findings are recorded in the dental record.

7. *Radiography.* Routine bite-wing radiographs should not be taken more than once a year. Vertical bite-wing views will provide a better picture of the alveolar bone and are preferred over standard bite-wings in periodontics. Full-mouth radiographs should be taken whenever

DATE_____

□ REEVAL   □ POST TREATMENT EVAL   □ MAINTENANCE EVAL

(1) Med Hx: □ Change. □ No change. ALERT:_____

(2) Oral Mucosal Tissue:_____

(3) Gingival Tissue:_____

(4) Pockets—4mm   (5) Bleeding sites—circle red   (6) Mobility—I, II, III   (7) Caries   (8) Plaque—blue

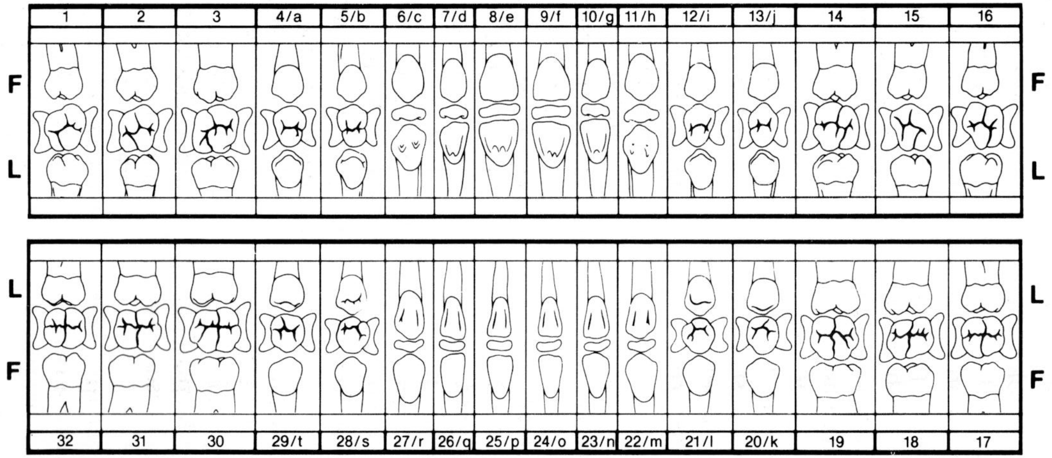

F																L
1	2	3	4/a	5/b	6/c	7/d	8/e	9/f	10/g	11/h	12/i	13/j	14	15	16	

L																F
32	31	30	29/t	28/s	27/r	26/q	25/p	24/o	23/n	22/m	21/l	20/k	19	18	17	

Bleeding Score_____   Plaque Score_____

Prophy: Category I II III IV

(9) Treatment Received:_____

Future Recommendations

Prognosis:_____

Personalized Tr:_____

Time:_____ With:_____ Est. Fee:_____ Signature:_____ Interval:_____ Category Prophy:_____

Fig. 24—1.

required, but seldom more frequently than every 3 years.

8. *Plaque evaluation.* After the entire clinical examination has been performed, a plaque evaluation is completed. The sequencing is important, because the dyes usually used in plaque detection will color the teeth and especially the soft tissue, making clinical examination difficult. All sites with plaque present can be recorded on an oral hygiene chart and the plaque index is then calculated. The oral hygiene chart will show areas that patients have difficulty in cleaning. The plaque index can be used to demonstrate to patients how well they are performing plaque-control procedures.

THERAPEUTIC PROCEDURES

1. Routine Maintenance Therapy

a. *Oral hygiene instructions.* Oral hygiene instruction is tailored to the individual needs of each patient. Some patients always need reinforcement and encouragement. Refer to Chapter 6 for a discussion of plaque control.

b. *Scaling.* All interproximal and subgingival areas must be thoroughly debrided. Areas of deepened pockets require actual planing. Refer to Chapter 7 for a discussion on root preparation.

c. *Polishing.* Almost all plaque and stain can be removed with a polishing cup. A relatively new instrument, Prophyjet, removes plaque and stain by spraying a solution or paste of water and sodium bicarbonate crystals on the clinical crown of the tooth. The abrasive action of this instrument appears to be helpful in removing plaque and stain from supragingival surfaces. If used injudiciously, it may remove cementum

and dentin from an exposed root surface.

2. Adjuncts to Maintenance Therapy

a. *Fluoride use.* There are two forms.

(1) Fluoride preparation irrigation. A 1.64% solution of stannous fluoride has been shown to decrease significantly the percentages of spirochetes and motile rods in periodontal pockets. Placing stannous fluoride subgingivally, by means of an irrigation syringe, has the potential of reducing microorganisms that may have been left behind after root planing of deep crevices.

(2) Topical fluorides. These are applied by brushing or in trays to control caries and plaque.

b. *Periodontal surgery.* Occasionally, surgical therapy may be required as part of the periodontal maintenance phase. There should be no reluctance on the part of the dentist to recommend a surgical procedure that is clearly needed to extend the life of the dentition.

c. *Systemic antibiotic use.* A small percentage of patients do not respond to periodontal therapy. Systemic antibiotic therapy may be indicated in these patients to bring the disease under control. There is evidence to show that tetracycline and minocycline, a semisynthetic derivative of tetracycline, may be effective in controlling refractive cases of periodontitis. The dose of tetracycline is 250 mg every 6 hours for 14 days. The dose of minocycline is 200 mg per day for 2 weeks. In addition, some studies have demonstrated that metronidazole is useful against the gram-negative anaerobic bacteria and spirochetes associated with advanced periodontitis. The dosage of this drug is 250 mg, three times per day, for 3 to 7 days. Thorough local therapy must accompany the administration of systemic antibiotics. If plaque and calculus are not removed, the disease will not be brought under control. The potential for developing resistant bacterial strains as well as the systemic side-effects of repeated or long-term use of antibiotics, must be weighed against the potential benefits.

EFFECT OF AN EXCELLENT MAINTENANCE PROGRAM ON TOTAL DENTAL HEALTH

Six years of data from studies performed in Sweden showed that a thorough maintenance program, performed every 2 to 3 months, was capable of stabilizing periodontal disease in an adult population. The effect of this maintenance program on caries reduction was also impressive. The group on the frequent, regular maintenance program had 61 times less caries experience than the control group. There is no doubt that the maintenance aspect of therapy is a valuable and effective service for dental patients. Maintenance deserves the highest priority in the daily practice of dentistry.

Index

Numbers followed by *f* indicate figures; those followed by *t* indicate tables